HEALING WITH FIRE

CHÖGYAL NAMKHAI NORBU

HEALING *with* FIRE
A Practical Manual of Tibetan Moxibustion

Original Title in Tibetan
Me gtsa'i lag len nyung bsdus dwangs shel me long
The Clear Crystal Mirror
A Concise Guide to the Practice of Moxibustion

Translated and introduced by
Elio Guarisco

Edited by
Susan Schwarz

ཤང་ཞུང་དཔེ་སྐྲུན་ཁང་།
Shang Shung Publications

© 2011 Shang Shung Institute
58031 Arcidosso (GR)
Italy
www.shangshungpublications.org
info@shangshunginstitute.org

Cover design: Daniel Zegunis, Daria Grekova, and Denis Berezovskyi
Cover model: Alexandra Lubentsova
Cover photo: Alexandra Lubentsova and Ekaterina Shmarova
Graphic design: Daniel Zegunis and Anastasia Ermilova
Drawings: Tanita Ferrari
Point placement: Alexey Polionov
Plate layout: Grzegorz Niedzielski (Artismedia)
Flame symbol from a woodcut of Dorje Legpa (artist unknown) reproduced courtesy of Prima Mai
Chart in Appendix A, note 6, reproduced courtesy of John Eskenazi and Sam Fogg

ISBN 978-88-7834-113-5
IPC 641EN10
Approved by the International Publications Committee of the Dzogchen Community founded by Chögyal Namkhai Norbu

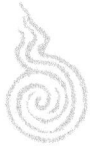

Contents

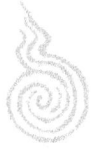

About This Book

Over the course of many years, Prof. Chögyal Namkhai Norbu has conducted an extensive comparative study of ancient manuals on moxibustion from the Tibetan medical tradition. The study is an ongoing process that is expected to culminate in the compilation of a manual classifying more than three thousand moxa points including the conditions they treat.

The present book is a practical summary presenting five hundred of the most important and useful moxa points with their indications. The author has prepared this condensed and essential guide in response to the need of those wishing to cultivate immediate knowledge of this ancient and valid method of healing.

Prof. Chögyal Namkhai Norbu is recognized around the world for his vast knowledge of Tibetan culture, including ancient Tibetan history and astrology, Tibetan spiritual paths such as Dzogchen and Vajrayana Buddhism, and traditional medicine. Trained in Tibetan medicine under exceptional teachers such as Rigdzin Changchub Dorje, Kyabje Kangkar Rinpoche, and Khenpo Khyenrab Chökyi Öser, he is considered an eminent authority and an unparalleled source of ancient knowledge such as the material presented here.[1]

Moxa is a relatively simple and extremely useful therapy. With due care, and paying attention to all of the precautions and safety measures explained in this manual, the two milder levels of moxa can be practiced even by those not trained in the various aspects of Tibetan medicine.

ABOUT THE TRANSLATION

This manual has been translated from Tibetan into English with the kind assistance of the author, who spent many hours with the translator clarifying the precise location of points and the nature of symptoms described in the text.

Wherever possible, the indications, some of which are specific to Tibetan medicine, have been rendered in terminology that is readily understandable for the reader. The book is intended for anyone wishing to study or apply moxa, from laypersons to skilled medical professionals.

It should be remembered that some of the expressions used to describe indications reflect concepts found in Tibetan traditional medicine that occasionally diverge from Western ideas.

Very general indications listed under the individual points, such as "stiffness," should be understood as applying to any part of the body. An index of indications makes it easier to identify which points can be used to treat individual conditions. Notes, some citing comments by the author and others added by the translator, have been provided to supplement the information in the book.

Drawings illustrating the position of the points have been included to facilitate the identification of their location. We are grateful to Tanita Ferrari for her sensitive renderings.

Susan Schwarz edited the English manuscript with great dedication and thoroughness, and her witty insights helped improve the overall structure. Without her assistance this book would still be a work in progress.

Nancy Simmons, English editor of Shang Shung Publications, reviewed the final manuscript in her usual meticulous and all-embracing way.

Dr. Phuntsog Wangmo, Director of the Shang Shung Institute School of Tibetan Medicine in Conway, Massachusetts, patiently and kindly offered valuable advice regarding the understanding and translation into English of various indications mentioned in the book.

Moreover, the translation and publication of this book has been made possible through the dedicated efforts of Oliver Leick, Director of Shang Shung Institute Austria, who arranged the financial support for the translation work.

Our thanks also go to the editorial staff of Shang Shung Publications for their support and collaboration, and, finally, to the many other people who freely and generously contributed their time and resources to bring this project to fruition.

The Translator

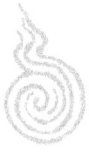

Translator's Introduction

TIBETAN MOXIBUSTION

THE ORIGIN OF MOXA

A widespread form of traditional healing in the East, moxibustion is one of the most ancient methods of healing. Although often erroneously referred to as a Chinese therapy, much evidence shows that this is not the case. Moxibustion was practiced in Shang Shung, a kingdom whose existence can be traced back almost four thousand years.[1] It was the cradle of Tibetan civilization, with Mount Kailash as its center and heart. It is possible, however, that a rudimentary form of moxa existed in an even earlier period.

In the Tibetan language, moxa is referred to as *me btsa'* or, as written in the more ancient Shang Shung language, *me gtsa'*. Both spellings are pronounced *metsa*. *Me* means fire and *btsa'* focal point. The modern term moxa may well have derived from the Tibetan *metsa*.[2]

We assume that the technique of applying moxa underwent various changes over the course of time. Since primitive people used heated stones on the body to alleviate pain, it is plausible that later, with the discovery of metals such as iron, gold, and silver, these materials were also adopted as instruments for applying moxa. With the discovery of the medicinal properties of plants, these, too, were burned on the body. A variety of materials are still used today to transfer heat to the body, including stone, wood, horn, metal, and herbs.

This experiential knowledge evolved over the ages, and, from the eighth century onward, Tibetan medicine absorbed and integrated theories and methods of medical traditions imported from neighboring countries such as Persia, India, Nepal, and China. While in its rudimentary form moxa was applied only on general areas of the body, as knowledge of specific points with particular indications for their usage developed, the treatment of points located by measurement was gradually adopted as well.

TRADITIONAL CLIMATIC CONDITIONS FOR MOXA

Moxa is classically used for the prevention and treatment of illnesses caused by cold and humidity. As a heating and tonifying therapy, this method is therefore especially suited for the colder regions of the world, and hence more common there.

However, moxa can be used for a variety of problems in any geographic area, regardless of the climate. In hot seasons or locations, before applying moxa it is advisable to have the patient take a cold shower to make the body more receptive to heat.

HOW MOXA WORKS

Moxa is a therapy that uses the direct application of heat on areas of the body affected by a pathology, and in particular on specific points.

The nerve fibers of the skin represent a complex system receptive and responsive to stimuli. The skin, as the organ of touch, is one of the first recipients of external information entering our body and mind complex. In particular, the skin is equipped with thermoreceptors that convey heat stimuli to various other parts of the body and especially to the brain.

In addition, heat directly and indirectly reaches the flesh, the bones, and the organs through various aspects of our nervous system. Initially, the heat from the application of moxa constricts the blood vessels, but after a while the opposite reaction occurs, a process known as vasodilation. Moreover, when heat is applied for a long time, toxins in the tissues are dispersed, producing an anti-irritating effect. Finally, the body contains energetic pathways and centers, not necessarily identical to those used in Chinese acupuncture, through which heat can release its healing power.

Moxa works directly by infusing heat to organs and parts of the body, and indirectly by conveying information to these organs and parts of the body through the nervous system and through subtle and less obvious energetic pathways that interact with the brain, nerves, and all the bodily constituents.

THERAPEUTIC BENEFITS OF MOXA

Since moxa is principally a method of infusing the body with the energy of heat, it is particularly indicated when heat decreases and the cold nature of Phlegm energy[3] increases in the body. An increase in the cold nature affects digestive heat first of all.

Digestive heat is the very basis for good health. Good digestive heat infuses the body with inner and outer radiance and confers a sharp intelligence, a strong determination in activities, and a long life. For these reasons, it is crucial to maintain good digestive heat, for instance, by eating foods that are easy to digest, exercising regularly, and taking herbs that strengthen digestive heat.

When digestive heat diminishes and symptoms such as flatulence, vomiting, or diarrhea manifest, foods are not properly digested and as a result either nutritional essence is depleted or nonassimilated nutritional essence is accumulated. In particular, the accumulation of residual nutritional essence in the organism can impair the self-regeneration process of the various parts of the body.

This condition favors the appearance of minor and major pathologies that manifest externally or internally. Internal conditions range from chronic indigestion to abdominal pain, nausea and vomiting, low body temperature, deficient blood circulation, tumors, edemas, neuralgia, lung disorders, and calculi. External conditions include rheumatism, arthritis, problems in the joints, and swellings.

In all of these cases, the regular application of moxa reduces the symptoms of the illness and helps the healing process.

In today's society we are witnessing a progressive increase in unhealthy lifestyles, paralleled by a loss of real values. Selfishness, worries, discontent with ourselves, fear, and expectations are just a few of the many attitudes that dominate our lives. In addition to physical illnesses, these attitudes, combined with the stressful pace to which we subject ourselves and the chemical-laden food we eat, are the source of many emotional disorders, known in Tibetan medicine as Wind energy disorders.[4]

These disorders manifest with symptoms such as sadness, insomnia, nervousness, excitement, depression, isolation, refusal to communicate, or lack of concentration and memory. Untreated, they can easily develop into emotional instability and serious illnesses such as schizophrenia and other psychoses.

Since the causes of these disorders are manifold, they should be addressed with a multi-pronged strategy that can include dietary changes, a different social environment, the administration of medicines when necessary, and the reestablishment of the basic ground of sanity through increased contact with the body.

Although it is obvious that the best remedy in these cases would be for the person to regain deeper values, regular application of moxa on the specific points indicated for these disorders can be a valid and strong support for other therapies.

As will be explained in this manual, moxa can be used to treat a wide variety of physical and emotional conditions.

WHEN MOXA IS NOT INDICATED

A general rule is that problems presenting a strong inflammatory condition should not be treated with moxa. In Tibetan medicine, these problems are referred to as Bile energy illnesses or acute conditions. For example, a sprain or a painful and swollen ankle cannot be treated with moxa, nor can conditions in which the patient does not tolerate heat and has fixed, acute pain.

However, some problems related to Bile energy can be treated with moxa, for instance digestive problems arising due to the slow release of bile liquid. In such cases, moxa can help activate the bile and improve the digestion.[5]

Fevers that have been caused by trauma, or in which an emotional condition plays a major role, as well as persistent low-grade fevers or fevers in their conclusive stage, can be treated with moxa, provided the temperature of the patient does not exceed 38 °C (100.4 °F).

Moxa is generally not indicated for blood disorders either, as heat may aggravate the problem. However, moxa can be used effectively to ameliorate poor blood circulation and release blood congestion in a specific area of the body. Also, if applied on the right points, the cauterization method of direct application that leaves scar tissue can reduce high blood pressure in that it reduces the thickness of blood and has a vasodilatory effect.

Given these factors, it is important to ascertain the general cold or hot nature of a patient's disorder before electing moxa as an appropriate form of treatment.

METHODS OF APPLYING MOXA

The prevalent method of applying moxa in Tibet in the past was quite radical. The tip of metal instruments called *tel* and *tsug*[6] was heated in a fire and applied directly on the point when red hot, cauterizing the skin and causing a major burn with consequent scarring.

In addition to this extreme method, called cauterization, Tibetan medical texts describe three other modes of applying moxa: burning, heating, and threatening. Each is characterized by a descending degree of heat intensity and a recommended number of applications. Each of these methods, as explained in Part One, is indicated for specific types of disease and different categories of people. Only the first two methods entail a certain degree of burning the skin.

In present-day society, the most extreme method, involving cauterization and scarring, is rarely employed since physical appearance is considered important and pain is generally avoided whenever possible. Moreover, according to the author of this book, milder forms of moxa can yield the same results as the stronger ones without burning and wounding the skin.

For children, the elderly, persons with a nervous disposition, and pregnant women, it is advisable to apply the mildest form of moxa, called threatening.

ARTEMISIA

Today, the most common method of applying moxa therapy is to burn an herb compressed into cones or sticks on or near specific points on the body. Cones are one of the most effective ways of generating heat, while sticks are easier to use.

Although Tibetan practice favors a high-altitude plant in the same genus as the edelweiss, the herb most prevalent in moxibustion therapy today is artemisia, another genus belonging to the daisy or *Asteraceae* family.[7] Artemisia can be found in temperate climates throughout the world. The principal species used is *Artemisia verlotiorum* (Chinese mugwort), often confused with the less aromatic *A. vulgaris* or common mugwort. *Artemisia abrotanum, A. princeps,* and *A. capillaris* are also used.

Artemisia has tonic, febrifugal, antiepileptic, emmenagogic, and nervine properties as well as the special quality of balancing the bodily constituents.

Harvesting and processing artemisia oneself may prove unnecessarily complicated as ready-to-use moxa wool, known also as moxa punk, is available from most acupuncture suppliers. Technically, the term moxa refers to the wool, while the word moxibustion connotes the therapeutic use of moxa.

Artemisia can be used alone or mixed with other herbs according to the problem to be treated. However, the main therapeutic action is performed by the heat.[8]

MAKING MOXA CONES

To prepare cones, press a piece of moxa wool in the palm of your hand with the thumb until it becomes compact. Compacting the herb helps produce more heat and makes it easier for the heat to penetrate more deeply. Then shape it into a cone tapering to a small tip for easy ignition.

Alternatively, use a piece of rolling paper to compact the moxa into an oval "cigarette," shaped like a candy in a wrapper twisted at each end, cutting it in half to make two moxa cones. If the paper is thin enough, it can be burned with the cone. Otherwise it can be carefully removed so the cone retains its shape. Yet another method to compact the moxa is to cut off the corner of an unpleated plastic bag, press the moxa into the corner, twist it, and then untwist it to release the compressed cone. The images on page 4 illustrate the process of making cones.

Moxa cones can vary in size depending on the part of the body where they will be applied, the type of problem to be treated, and the age of the patient.

For the spine and the back, the cones should be somewhere between the size of the last phalanx of the patient's little finger and a bit larger than the last phalanx of the index finger. When applied on the head, neck, chest, abdomen, and limbs, the cones should be smaller, about the size of the last phalanx of the little finger. For children, the cones should be the size of a pea. Moxa "grains" about the size of a barley seed can be used on the joints of the fingers.

In special cases, such as the treatment of benign tumors, the cones need to be bigger, about the size of the last phalanx of the patient's thumb. To relieve shooting pains, the cones should be flatter.

Since they burn longer and produce more heat, larger cones can be used for people with a strong constitution or when stronger heat stimulation is needed.

On delicate areas of the body, such as the face, or when a large area of the body is affected or sore, it is more suitable to use moxa sticks instead of applying cones directly to the skin. This method makes it easier to calibrate the infusion of heat on the point and allows for the treatment of larger areas.

Ready-made Japanese or Korean cones are a valid substitute for manually prepared moxa cones. These small cones or tubes of compacted artemisia have an adhesive round paper base with a hole in the center, which allows heat to be conducted to the point.

DIRECT MOXA WITH CONES

In the direct moxa method, the cone is applied directly on the surface of the skin. The patient should sit or lie down in a position that facilitates the application of the cones. When placing each cone, it is important to ensure that it remains stable. If the cone does not readily rest on the area of application, the point can be dampened with garlic or ginger juice so that the cone will adhere to the skin and not fall off.

The heat transferred to a part of the body or point needs to be constant. To achieve this effect, apply one cone after the other in succession. Just before the first cone is ready to be removed (depending on the degree of heat called for in the treatment), light another cone so that it is already burning when applied. With practice, you will develop a sense for timing the process of replacing one cone with the next. Since the cones ignite easily, it is sufficient to touch them with a lit stick of incense. You might find a lighter or matches too difficult to control.

Direct moxa can be used for cauterization and burning, in which case the cones are burned down to the skin with repeated applications and the heat leaves a mark of varying degrees. This technique can be useful in cases where fluid needs to be drained or an inflammation or infection blocked inside needs to be released. If a blister appears, the area is cleaned with cold boiled water and an appropriate antiseptic oil is applied. Traditionally, in Tibet salted butter was used. If suppuration occurs, the area needs daily cleaning and antiseptic oil applied around the rim of the scar until it heals. This technique of burning the skin is not advisable unless there is a real necessity since it requires considerable skill on the part of the practitioner. If this latter method is used on hairy parts of the body, the hair around the point should first be shaved.

Direct moxa is also suitable for milder treatments, in which case the cones are removed before they have burned completely to avoid harming the skin.

INDIRECT MOXA WITH CONES

In the indirect method, a base or support is placed under the cone so there is no direct contact with the surface of the skin. It can be used for burning, heating, and threatening.

In the case of Wind energy disorders, paralysis, or abscesses, place the cone on a slice of garlic. For Phlegm energy disorders, use a slice of ginger. A thin layer of wood also serves as an appropriate base. Traditionally, berberis wood is used.

Whichever material you choose, to allow the heat to penetrate, make small holes all over the base with a needle and a larger hole in the center.

When using the indirect method, take care to remove the base as soon as the sensation of heat becomes too strong as you might otherwise burn the patient. The base should be changed after about five cone applications.

Other substances can also serve as a base for cones, including sea salt, ground herb paste, and clay. Each has specific indications. When treating the point in the navel, for instance, you can fill the cavity with salt and place the cone either directly on the salt or on another support. This method of indirect moxa can also be effective when the heat is generated with a moxa stick.

When treating hairy parts of the body, separate the hair, pressing it down with the index and middle fingers spread apart; then let the heat from the stick pass between the two fingers. Alternatively, in treatments with cones, use a wooden spoon, with a central hole a little smaller than the base of the cone or many smaller holes, as a support.

MOXA STICKS

Although moxa cones are considered to have a stronger effect than moxa sticks, the sticks are easier to use. Furthermore, sticks are ideal for treating delicate and sensitive areas of the body, such as the ears, around the eyes, the nose, and other parts of the face, and in proximity to glands and veins or arteries. They are also advisable when the main purpose of treatment is tonification.

Several types of sticks or rolls are readily available. The most common are made of compressed moxa wrapped in paper, in which instance the outer label should be peeled back before use. Another type, referred to as smokeless moxa, is made of compressed charcoal with powdered artemisia.

There are various methods of application. One is to hold the stick perpendicular to the point, gradually bringing the burning tip closer to the skin and then keeping it at about three-quarters of an inch (two centimeters) from the point. As soon as the patient indicates that the heat has become too strong to tolerate, retract the stick a little to give relief to the patient and after a few moments bring it close again. When you hold the stick close to the point, rest your hand on the body of the patient, if possible, so as to maintain stability.

In another method, referred to as pecking, slowly bring the stick close to the point, retract it slowly, and then bring it closer again in steady alternation.

To transfer heat to a larger area, keep the stick at a distance of about three-quarters of an inch from the skin and make slow rotary movements with its tip over the area, as if tracing a looped flower pattern that overlaps in the center. Use this method to tonify areas such as knee joints affected by cold or pain.

When ash forms, roll it off the tip of the stick to prevent it from falling on the patient and to allow the proper emission of heat. At the end of the session, extinguish the stick by wrapping its tip in tinfoil or inserting it in ash or sand.

THE NATURE OF THE MOXA POINTS

The Tibetan moxa therapy presented in this manual is applied on localized areas of the body as well as on specific points. The points in this system of moxa coincide only partially with traditional Chinese acupuncture points, including those found on the meridians.

Moxa can be applied on various parts of the body where particular pathologies manifest, such as pain, non-inflammatory swellings, and the retention of fluids. We have referred to these areas as localized points.

In such cases, the heat of moxa works locally in unblocking the Wind energy, Phlegm energy, and blood that may be blocked in the skin, flesh, organs, nerves, tendons, ligaments, and bones.

But the most fascinating, and sometimes unexpected in terms of the indications they treat, are the fixed points located by measurement. Their therapeutic benefits have been known in the East for millennia. The fixed points identified in ancient moxibustion manuals are found throughout the body – on the back, front, head, arms, legs, hands, and feet – and can be used to treat specific conditions.

Many of these points were presumably recognized in ancient times on the basis of special knowledge of the subtle energetic structure of the human organism.

In addition to the visible muscular, vascular, nervous, and lymphatic system, the body has a subtle and less detectable network of energies, pathways of energies, and vital essences.

Many of the fixed moxa points appear to be located on an energetic structure connecting the internal hollow and solid organs, the senses, and the Wind, Bile, and Phlegm energies that govern all physiological functions.

By applying moxa on these points, we can work on the physical problems as well as on the energetic level underlying the arising of imbalances and diseases.

POINTS ON THE BACK

The points along the spine, and in particular those on the vertebrae, appear to have a slightly different nature and function than the points on the front of the body.

These points are located along the spinal cord that tapers downward within the spinal cavity from its source in the brain. The peripheral nervous system composed of major and minor nerves is connected with the spinal cord. Among the major nerves, sensory nerves conduct stimuli and motor nerves stimulate muscular contraction.

The minor nerves comprise the autonomic nervous system, which according to Tibetan medicine carries Wind energy to the heart; Bile energy to the lungs, large intestine, liver, and gallbladder; Phlegm energy to the stomach, spleen, kidneys, and bladder; and all three energies to the male and female reproductive organs.

Since the moxa points on the spine are located where the nerve roots directly associated with the internal organs exit the spinal cord, these points are effective for treating chronic and tenacious conditions of the respective organs.

The first moxa point on the spine corresponds to the seventh cervical vertebra. Treatment on this point can be very effective in alleviating deep-seated emotional and mental problems. Moxa on the second vertebra, the equivalent of the first thoracic, effectively counteracts weak Bile energy function. Treatment on the third vertebra alleviates general cold conditions.

The following vertebrae, up to and including the eighteenth, are connected to specific organs and are thus used primarily for treating the related pathologies.

The points on the sixth and seventh vertebrae are connected to the coronaries and heart respectively, and in addition to the corresponding pathologies are also used for treating emotional and mental problems. This is because the heart and coronaries are the main seat of life energy, which when unbalanced affects the mind of the person.

This manual lists four spinal points located on the sacrum and one on the tailbone. All are connected to the Wind energy governing the functions of the sexual organs and the expulsion of urine, feces, and menstrual blood.

Above the seventh cervical, there are several moxa points described in the extraordinary, visionary medical instructions of Rigdzin Changchub Dorje.[9]

Moxa on the cervical points can treat bacterial diseases of the nose, ears, teeth, and head; Wind energy and Blood disorders affecting the head; and neurological problems caused by exposure to external negative influences.

The points on the lateral back have somewhat mixed indications. A series of points found only in the instructions of Rigdzin Changchub Dorje is located on the back of the shoulder, an area traversed by many nerves that descend into the arms.

These points on the shoulders are used to treat esophageal obstruction caused by gastric reflux, cardiac pains, mysterious energetic connections that are hard to assess, and neurological illnesses resulting from exposure to negative influences and provocations.

Moxa on other points on the lateral back relieves pain and problems of motility of the shoulders and arms. A series of other points is located right above organs such as lungs, heart, stomach, liver, spleen, and kidneys; these points are used in the treatment of a variety of disorders affecting these organs.

Underscoring the connection between the lungs and the lower digestive apparatus, and in particular the large intestine, some points located near the lungs are also used to treat intestinal problems.

POINTS ON THE FRONT

The points on the front of the body are directly connected to the nerve network stemming from the brain and the spinal cord and to energetic pathways. This is why many of these points, particularly those on the neck and immediately below it, are related to treatment of a variety of different illnesses ranging from nosebleed to tuberculosis, from high blood pressure to depressive syndrome.

However, many of the front points are located right above various important regions and organs, such as the lungs, heart, epigastrium, digestive system, and the genito-urinary system. Accordingly, moxa applied on the front of the body acts to relieve the immediate pathologies of these organs as well as those that have become chronic. Treatment of these points is especially effective for swift relief of the symptoms of stomach, lung, heart, and intestinal problems.

Located in sensitive areas of the body, the points on the front of the torso must be treated with particular care, using smaller cones of moxa as mentioned above.

POINTS ON THE EXTREMITIES

In the Tibetan language, the extremities[10] include not only the arms and legs but also the head, the most important extremity.

The points on the head are particularly significant for a varied range of therapeutic applications. They begin at the crown of the head, a sensitive area at the juncture of the cranial bones along the sagittal suture. The point on the crown is often treated with a special method known as golden needle therapy in which a twenty-four-carat gold needle is inserted in the skin above the skull with a ball of moxa affixed at the top. While the moxa burns, its healing properties pass from the needle to the entire body. This method is considered especially effective for epilepsy and a number of other hard-to-cure diseases.

In addition to minor cerebral problems, the points on the head are useful in the treatment of cranial bone pain and all complaints manifesting in connection with the head, face, and sense organs (eyes, ears, and nose). They are also beneficial for curing forgetfulness, impaired mental functions, and emotional and mental conditions.

Three points on the skull, known as cranial suture points,[11] have a particular function. Located on the anterior fontanel on the frontal bone, the crown of the head on the parietal bone, and the lambdoid suture, they are twelve, sixteen, and twenty finger-widths from the tip of the nose, respectively, on a straight line to the center of the occipital bone. All are useful in cases of dizziness, epilepsy, and dazed sensations.

Because of their location, the points on the upper arms can be used principally to treat pulmonary disorders as well as problems with the motility of neck, shoulder, and arms and blood problems in the upper body.

The points on the forearms, hands, and fingers are also connected to various parts of the body through vascular and energetic pathways and are thus effective for treating symptoms and diseases manifesting in other parts of the body as well, such as vomiting, nosebleed, problems related to the eyes, ears, and teeth, and other nonlocal conditions.

Similar to the arms, the points on the upper and lower parts of the legs support therapies treating malfunctions in the lower body (lower abdomen, waist, lumbar and sacral regions) and the legs. Because of their location on particular vascular and energy pathways, some points on the legs are effective in the treatment of constipation, infertility, gynecological disorders, digestive and urinary problems, and even weak eyesight. In particular, several points on the upper and lower legs and feet are used to treat various disorders of the male and female reproductive systems.

Moxa at the base of the heel and where hair grows on the big toe is also effective against insanity and seizures.

On both the legs and the feet, moxa can be applied to cure an accumulation of fluids in the joints in those parts of the body. These fluids are known as *chuser* in Tibetan medical terminology.[12] *Chuser* is a pale yellow, viscous fluid, the result of the process of refining the blood from the nutriment in the liver. Its primary location is in the joints and between the skin and flesh. *Chuser* is also present throughout various parts of the body such as the solid and hollow organs.

In this book, the term *chuser* has been translated as lymph. Most of the indications that refer to lymphatic disorders found throughout this manual should be understood to refer to fluids that accumulate predominantly in the locations just mentioned.

MEASURING POINTS

To measure the points on the spine, you first need to identify the first vertebra according to the Tibetan system of counting. Corresponding to the seventh cervical, it is easily recognizable since it is the most prominent bone on the back of the neck.[13]

When treating points on the backbone, moxa is applied on the spinous process of the vertebrae, not in between the vertebrae as this could cause damage to the nerves. Most of the points on the vertebrae are triple points, consisting of a central point on the spinous process, one a thumb to the left, and one a thumb to the right of the central one. As explained in Part One, a thumb in this context is a unit of measurement corresponding to the distance from the last joint of the thumb to the tip of the nail, always based on the patient's proportions.[14]

Moxa can be applied to all three points simultaneously, or, if the heat is deemed too strong, first on the central point, then the point on the patient's right, and finally the point on the left.[15]

To find the vertebrae, feel the spine of the patient with the thumb counting the vertebrae. Often, if the patient is overweight or has some abnormalities in the spine, it is not easy to locate the vertebrae. In that case, mark the length of a thumb unit (as described above) on a piece of string or paper and use this to measure the distance from the spinous process of one vertebra to the next. Remember, however, that the dorsal vertebrae are just short of a thumb apart, while the distance between the lumbar vertebrae is just over a thumb.

Other parts of the body, such as bones, can also be used as a reference to determine the position of individual vertebrae. For instance, the fourth vertebra in the Tibetan system (Posterior Lung Lobe Point; equivalent to T3) is at the same level as the medial part of the scapular spine. The eighth vertebra (Diaphragm Point; T7) is at the level of the inferior angle of the scapula. The seventeenth vertebrae (Small Intestine Point; L4) is at the level of the highest point of the iliac crest and the twentieth (Downward-Clearing Wind Point; S2) is at the level of the posterior superior iliac spine, further identified by the dimple on the lower back.

BEFORE, DURING, AND AFTER TREATMENT

As mentioned above, in hot climates or weather it is advisable to have the patient take a cold shower before treatment to help cool the body temperature.

Prior to treatment, have the patient lie down and relax. In general, moxa should not be applied right after meals. Ventilate the room both before and after treatment so that smoke from the burning moxa does not make the patient dizzy or nauseous or irritate the eyes and lungs.

Before applying moxa, check the area or point you want to treat. An area or point is suitable for moxa if pressure with the thumb produces an indentation or pain, but also when pressure alleviates existing pain. Another sign of suitability is if the area or point is cold to the touch, swollen, and insensitive, generally indicating an imbalance of Phlegm energy. Finally, itchiness of a point or an area generally indicates an imbalance of Wind energy and hence confirms its appropriateness for treatment.

If strong heat is felt upon palpating the area or point, the area or point should be considered unsuitable for moxa treatment at that particular time. Also examine the skin of the patient. If the skin appears to be delicate, thin, or wrinkled in the area where you want to apply moxa, you should take particular care not to burn it.

After strong forms of moxa, press the point with your thumb and apply some salted butter or antiseptic cream to the point. After mild treatments, the points can be massaged lightly with oil. The patient should also be advised to follow the other guidelines recommended in Part One.[16] For instance, the patient should walk around a little after a session to reestablish the circulation of the energies in the body.

The heat infused may take as long as two days to reach the inner parts of the organs. Hence, after treatment it is important for the patient to avoid cold drinks and foods for the rest of the day and cold showers for the next few days.

NUMBER OF MOXA APPLICATIONS

The number of cones applied in a treatment session varies according to the problem to be treated and the method of application. Generally speaking, to infuse sufficient heat, apply five to seven cones of moxa per session to each point treated, and more if necessary.

When using sticks, the amount of time for treating a point should be roughly the same as if you were using cones.

In the methods requiring cauterizing or burning of the skin, explained in Part One, the general rule is to apply twenty-one and fifteen cones, respectively.

When the treatment is sufficient, the area or point should appear rosy and feel hot to the touch; the patient also may start to perspire. As another sign that the moxa application is sufficient, heat may be felt on the opposite side of the body.

A single session of moxa can be enough to relieve pain or cure a minor problem. For chronic or serious conditions, three, seven, or more sessions may be required with intervals of one to three days. In some cases, however, it is better leave intervals of a week before repeating treatment.

PRECAUTIONS REGARDING THE APPLICATION OF MOXA

Regardless whether you apply direct or indirect moxa, do not underestimate the potentially harmful qualities of heat. Always keep in mind that although some patients have a significantly higher tolerance for heat than others, this does not make their skin less susceptible to burning. It is good practice to make it clear to patients that their communication is crucial. Similarly, some people have very low tolerance and/ or more sensitive skin than others. In particular the first time you are working with a patient, apply extreme caution to avoid inadvertent burns. Once you understand his or her threshold, you can work within a broader range. Pay close attention to the coloring of the skin during application; for the burning, heating, and threatening methods, a slight rosiness of the treated area is a sign that a sufficient level of heating has been achieved.

With the exception of a few points specifically indicated in this manual, when applying moxa it is advisable to avoid glands, veins, arteries, and sense organs. If treatment is required in the proximity of sensitive areas such as these, it is better to choose the milder methods of infusing heat (heating and threatening) and apply a technique allowing for the accurate calibration of the heat transferred.

UNUSUAL INDICATIONS

The peculiarity from a Western point of view of some of the indications given for certain moxa points necessitates a few words of explanation.

According to Tibetan medicine and the ancient Tibetan culture, there are illnesses that arise as a result of a disturbance in an individual's energy. This concept entails a perception of reality that we do not commonly have in modern scientific thought, and yet people do unknowingly suffer from such problems.

From the perspective of ancient Tibetan tradition, life is energy, a force that interacts with the energy of the five elements. The energy of the five elements composing the body is known as the *la* in the Tibetan language, translated here as protective energy.[17] The *la* is the factor that serves as the bridge or link between the inner and outer world of an individual.

A person's protective energy can weaken as a result of various conditions, such as an accident or severe shock. The weakening is indicated by signs such as a wasted appearance, fear, physical and mental debility, and unhappiness.

As a result of the weakening of the protective energy, a person becomes exposed to external negative influences, both simple or dominated by certain types of beings that can manifest in the form of various illnesses, from neuralgia to paralysis, from simple malaise to cancer.

The sources of such illnesses are classified under the terms *drib*, translated here as contamination, and *dön*, as provocations.[18]

These illnesses are recognized by a pulse that is not uniform and changes frequently, at times quick, at times slow. Moreover, the pulse associated with a particular organ may be absent, while another pulse associated with a different organ may be irregular, stopping and starting in a jerking fashion. Such illnesses can also be diagnosed through the examination of urine and with astrological calculations.

In any event, the primary characteristic of illnesses caused by provocations is that they do not respond well to any kind of medicine or therapy.

The best method for those of us who cannot easily access the ancient Tibetan rituals used in such cases is to restore the protective energy through Yantra Yoga and other special methods that can be learned in authentic spiritual disciplines.[19] These methods are an indispensable support for moxa and any kind of therapy we may apply in such cases.

Tibetan Astrology and the Timing of Moxa Treatments

Based as it is on the close correlation between macrocosmic and microcosmic phenomena, Tibetan traditional medicine attaches considerable importance to astrological factors that may have an effect on a cure. Bearing little resemblance to Western astrology, the oldest branch of Tibetan astrology revolves around five elements and a twelve-year cycle intermeshing with other cycles of varying lengths.[20] It uses a lunar calendar that also makes distinctions between the days of the month and the hours of the day.

As is emphasized repeatedly in this manual, taking these factors into account could be crucial for the timing of strong therapies or procedures that can be referred to as invasive. In the case of moxibustion, only direct, cauterizing moxa falls into this category. The consideration of astrological aspects may also prove beneficial for the efficacy of external therapies or procedures of any kind.

Appendix A, Astrological Factors, gives detailed information on various astrological factors that can be of relevance for the timing of treatments and includes several charts facilitating the calculation of such factors.

Basic Principles of Tibetan Medicine

Most of the indications for the moxa points given in this manual are easily understood, but to fully grasp the meaning of a few, some knowledge of Tibetan medicine is required. Several basic principles are presented below with the intention of fostering such an understanding.

Macrocosm and Microcosm

According to Tibetan medicine, the universe is an aggregation of tiny particles, each containing the qualities and functions of four elements: earth, water, fire, and air. Interacting in the dimension of space, the element that is the base for all other elements, these four produce the entire macrocosm of the universe and the microcosm of beings.

The Three Energies

In the human body, the elements are seen as three different energies called Wind, Bile, and Phlegm. Wind, or *prana*, has the mobile quality of the air element. Bile has the hot quality of the fire element. Phlegm has the solid and stable qualities of the earth element and the moist and wet qualities of the water element.

These three energies are the bases for the formation, life, and destruction of the human body.

Wind

Wind energy is first and foremost the life force that is inseparable from the mind of the individual. It is both the air we breathe and our internal energy.

Residing in specific areas of the body such as the brain and nerves, heart and chest, digestive tract and anal region, as well as in the bones, Wind energy governs many functions of body and mind, in particular those having to do with motility.

Memory, awareness, sense perception, speech, physical movements, the generation of effort, the opening and closing of the orifices, the workings of the nervous system, and the circulation of the nutritive essence through blood all depend on Wind energy. Intellectual sharpness, excitement, and sexual pleasure, too, are conferred by this energy.

Bile

Bile energy predominantly refers to the heat present in all parts of the body as the base of the life force.

Residing in the digestive tract, liver, gallbladder, heart, blood, eyes, and skin, Bile energy has various functions; in particular, it regenerates all the bodily constituents and the blood.

Strength and courage in achieving personal aims, analytical judgment, a good complexion, good eyesight, digestive heat, proper metabolism, and bodily temperature all depend on Bile energy.

Phlegm

Phlegm energy represents primarily the humid and wet components of the organism, which have a cool nature.

Residing in the head, tongue, salivary glands, spleen, pancreas, chest, stomach, kidneys, bladder, and joints, Phlegm energy has various functions; in particular, it maintains the moisture the body needs and produces gastric juices.

Mental stability, the sense of satisfaction from sense perceptions, the experience of taste, the process of digesting food, and ease in movements and sleep all depend on Phlegm energy.

CONSTITUTIONAL TYPES

Depending on which of the three energies predominate, individuals have different psychophysical constitutions.

Persons with a Wind constitution have a slightly curved back, are thin and have weak physical strength, an unhealthy complexion, and an excess of desire. They are generally not liked by others. When they walk or move their joints creak. They are talkative and rough in character, sleep lightly, and cannot withstand cold. They like singing and laughing, but their lifespan is short and wealth limited. Moreover, their metabolism is irregular, at times quick and at times slow.

Persons with a Bile constitution have strong hunger and thirst and a yellowish complexion. They perspire profusely, have middling physical strength, a sharp intellect, and tend to be proud. They are enterprising and can be callous. Their lifespan and wealth are middling. Moreover, their body is hot, and they have a quick metabolism.

Persons with a Phlegm constitution are tall, endowed with great physical strength, are devoid of malice, and have a fair complexion. They walk with the back slightly bent backward, are relaxed, and have a good nature. Their character is stable. They withstand hunger and thirst and sleep heavily. Their lifespan is long and their wealth great. Moreover, their body is cold, and they have a slow metabolism.

Most individuals are a mixture of two or more of these constitutions; classic types tend to be rare. Persons in whom all three energies are present exhibit the best physical traits and personality and rarely get sick.

HOW IMBALANCES ARISE

Health, both physical and psychological, depends on the harmony and interaction of these energies. Various conditions can disrupt the balance of Wind, Bile, and Phlegm, such as diet, behavior, accidents, and provocations of energy.

As a consequence of such conditions, the three energies can become deficient, in excess, or in conflict with each other, provoking various illnesses of both body and mind. Tibetan medicine classifies illnesses in the three categories Wind, Bile, and Phlegm. Wind disorders manifest as a consequence of eating an excess of light, raw, and non-nutritious food; not eating or sleeping adequately; working on an empty stomach; having too much sex; being exposed to wind and cold; engaging in intense intellectual activity; and talking excessively. Grief, worries, and mental fixation related to attachment are particularly prone to provoke Wind conditions. Wind disturbances are aggravated in the summer, in the afternoon, and at dawn.

Bile disorders manifest as a consequence of eating an excess of pungent, hot, and oily food, in particular nutritious foods such as fatty meat, and drinking excessive amounts of alcohol; engaging in excessive physical activity such as hard manual labor and exercise; experiencing physical trauma; sleeping during the afternoon; and being exposed to heat and dryness. These disorders are aggravated in the autumn, at midday, and at midnight.

Phlegm disorders manifest as a consequence of eating too much sweet, oily, cool, and heavy food, getting too little physical exercise, sleeping during the daytime, living in humid places, and being exposed to cold. Particular contributing factors include inactivity related to mental passivity, the consumption of stale or raw food and dairy products, and not leaving sufficient time between meals. These disorders are aggravated in the spring, evening, and morning.

THE SYMPTOMS OF IMBALANCE

Imbalances of Wind energy can be recognized by the presence of restlessness, dimming of the senses, yawning, trembling, a recurrent need to stretch the limbs, cold shivering, aching hips, waist, and joints, acute shifting pains, nausea, and unproductive retching. On an empty stomach these symptoms are stronger. The tongue is red, dry, and coarse; the pulse is floating and disappears with pressure; and the urine has an azure tinge and big bubbles.

Imbalances of Bile energy can be recognized by the presence of a bitter taste in the mouth, headaches, hypothermia, and acute pain in the upper body. After digestion these symptoms are aggravated. The tongue is coated with pale yellow mucus; the pulse is rapid and tight; and the urine is orange and malodorous.

Imbalances of Phlegm energy are recognized by a loss of appetite, difficult digestion, vomiting, a sticky mouth, a sensation of abdominal fullness, belching, lassitude, apathy, and an inner and outer sensation of cold. After meals these symptoms are aggravated. The tongue is pale white, smooth, and moist; the pulse is sunken, weak, and slow; and the urine is transparent like water, with little odor and vapor.

FOUR LINES OF TREATMENT

Once the nature of an illness has been recognized, it needs to be treated with a multipronged approach starting with dietary and behavioral changes, the administration of medicines, and the application of external therapies. These four lines of treatment balance the three energies with deliberately opposite qualities.

Diet

Wind imbalances are somewhat reduced by introducing nutritious and oily foods to the diet, for instance aged meat, lamb, bone broth, marrow, gnocchi made of barley flour, rice soup, toasted barley soup, molasses, sesame oil, butter, garlic and onion, nutmeg, nuts, and aged ale.

Bile imbalances are reduced with foods having cooling or bitter qualities, such as meat of herbivorous game, goat meat, fresh cereal soups, millet soup, soups containing toasted barley flour, whole grain cereals, yoghurt, buttermilk, goat milk, soup made with turnip leaves or dandelion, sugar, and boiled cold water.

Phlegm disorders are reduced with foods having a warming quality such as mutton, pork, fish, honey, soup made with freshly toasted barley or strong cereals, peas, soy, salt, pepper, ginger, chili, ale, and boiled hot water.

Behavior

Joyful entertainment, the cultivation of an easygoing attitude, and dwelling in warm places are some of the behaviors that alleviate Wind imbalances.

Physical and mental relaxation and dwelling in cool places are among the behaviors that alleviate Bile imbalances.

Behaviors that alleviate Phlegm imbalances include activity, movement, physical exercise, yoga, and dwelling in warm places.

Medicines

Medicines to counteract imbalances of the three energies are based on ingredients whose tastes counteract the qualities of the energies themselves. These ingredients can be herbs, minerals, or other substances. Tibetan medicine uses a vast array of ingredients, prepared as decoctions, powders, pills, creams, and tonics.

External therapies

Of the four lines of treatment, the external therapies are the form that can have the quickest and strongest effect. They include bloodletting, moxa, medical baths, stone and compress therapy, and massage.

In brief, illnesses of a hot nature (acute illnesses) are treated with four cold types of treatment: a cold diet consisting of light and less nutritious foods; cold behavior, such as living in a cool climate; cold medicine such as camphor; and a cold treatment such as bloodletting.

Illnesses of a cold nature (chronic illnesses) are treated with four hot types of treatment: a hot diet consisting of warming and nutritious foods; hot behavior, such as living in a warm climate; hot medicines such as pomegranate; and a hot external therapy such as moxa.

Generally speaking, bloodletting is indicated for Bile imbalances; various forms of moxa are indicated for Wind and Phlegm imbalances; massage with oils for Wind imbalances; and medical baths for various energy imbalances.

MOXIBUSTION AS A COMPLEMENTARY THERAPY

Moxibustion's suitability as a therapy for chronic and complex conditions makes it a particularly valuable modality to supplement, and in some cases even replace, conventional methods of treatment. At once concise and comprehensive, the author's guidance brings unprecedented clarity to this profound and little known tradition, giving us the tools to use the natural power of heat as a means to unblock trapped energy so the process of healing can begin.

Homage

May all be auspicious!

I pay homage to my kind and wise medicine teachers
From the vast land of Tibet,
Khyenrab Öser, Shedrup Chökyi Senge, and Changchub Dorje,
Three manifestations of the King of Healing,
By composing this brief manual
On the external therapy of moxibustion.

PART ONE
Tibetan Moxibustion Therapy

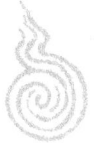

The Practice of Moxibustion

The Secret Oral Instruction Tantra, Essence of Nectar[1] and other texts explain the various forms of external therapies[2] and classify them into five types: bloodletting, moxibustion, medical baths, stone and compress therapy, and massage.[3] Among these external therapies, moxibustion brings consistently high benefits with few risks and is relatively easy to practice.

The essential principles of moxa practice as one of the five external therapies can be summarized in eight points:

1) How to Prepare Moxa
2) Cases in Which Moxa Is Indicated
3) Cases in Which Moxa Is Contraindicated
4) Types of Moxa Points
5) How to Locate Moxa Points
6) Methods of Applying Moxa
7) Post-Treatment Guidelines
8) Benefits of Moxa

Moxa practice should be learned through these eight points.

1) HOW TO PREPARE MOXA

Collect the appropriate herbs for moxa[4] on an auspicious day[5] during any of the three autumn months.[6] After beating the fresh plant to bruise the leaves,[7] place it to dry in the shade.[8] Once the herb is completely dry, remove its veins.[9] Adding a little charcoal powder from good quality softwood such as pine[10] will facilitate burning. Wrap the right quantity of herb prepared in this way in a piece of paper and press it into a firm lump.[11]

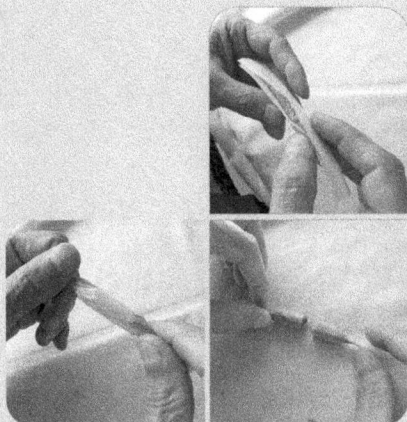

(1) Rice paper cones

For this style of cones, thin rice paper or cigarette paper holds the artemisia in place while burning.

Roll a small quantity of moxa in a piece of thin rice paper or large cigarette paper. The amount of moxa and size of the paper depend on the desired size of the cone.

Twist both ends like a candy wrapper.

Cut the "cigarette" in half to produce two cones. Placing the cone on the point to be treated, the twisted end is lit.

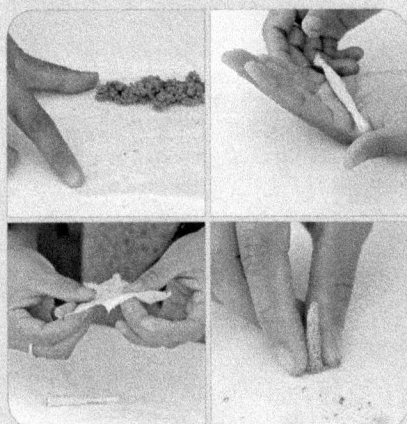

(2) Rice paper cones with paper removed

In this style of cone, rice paper is used as an aid to compress the cone, but is removed before burning.

Depending on the desired size of the cone, place a quantity of moxa on a piece of thin rice paper.

Roll a moxa "cigarette," pressing it between the palms repeatedly to compress the moxa, and twist both ends.

Cut the "cigarette" in half with a razor or sharp scissors and carefully remove the paper.

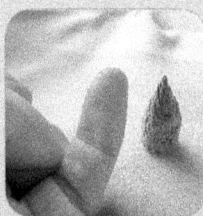

(3) Free-hand cones

Cones can also be made without paper, by compressing moxa in the palm of the hand.

Use the thumb to compress the moxa.

Again, the size of the finished cone depends on the point to be treated.

See Translator's Introduction, pages xiii and xiv.

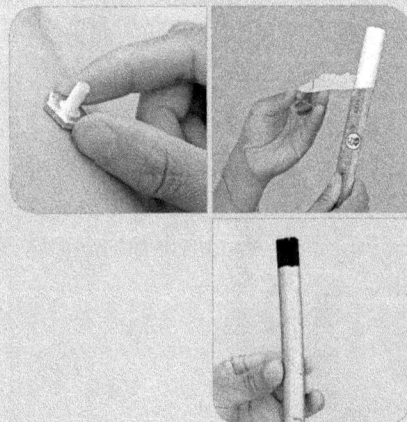

(4) Other forms of moxa

a. Self-adhesive Japanese style cones are made with a built-in support.

b. Chinese-style moxa rolls often have an outer paper wrapper that needs to be removed prior to lighting the roll.

c. "Smokeless" moxa rolls give off less smoke and odor.

For cases in which moxa needs to be applied directly, for example so as to cauterize the skin,[12] the lump of moxa should be made into a conical shape that is larger and more spherical in the center, with a thin and pointed tip so it can catch fire quickly. However, treatments requiring the direct, cauterizing application of moxa should only be performed by qualified doctors.

Nowadays, prefabricated moxa rolls, often made in China, are readily available and quite easy to use. The Japanese stick-on moxa cones are another popular form that is both easy to apply and very effective. In this method, small paper stick-on tubes containing compacted artemisia are placed on the appropriate point, producing the proper effect of moxa without the risk of injury from burns to the patient's body.[13]

2) CASES FOR WHICH MOXA IS INDICATED

The illnesses for which moxa is indicated include:

- Loss of metabolic heat[14]
- First-stage edema[15]
- Third-stage edema[16]
- Tumors[17]
- Cysts[18]
- Cold Bile illnesses[19]
- Lymphatic disorders[20]
- Poor digestion[21]
- Epigastric disorders[22]
- Chronic gastritis[23]
- Empty fever[24]
- Insanity[25]
- Epilepsy[26]
- Illnesses caused by provocations of energy[27]
- Neurological and vascular disorders[28]
- Gout[29]
- Arthritis, rheumatoid arthritis[30]
- Persistent, low-grade fever[31]
- Although bloodletting is contraindicated after moxa, most illnesses treated with bloodletting should be followed up with a moxa treatment
- Sudden wounds or injuries[32]
- Cysts, anthrax,[33] swellings, and warts[34] can be treated by applying moxa directly on the location where the problem manifests

In summary, moxa is the best treatment for all illnesses of a cold nature deriving from Phlegm and Wind and for all neurological and lymphatic illnesses.

3) Cases for Which Moxa Is Contraindicated

There are three specific cases for which moxa is contraindicated:

a) Specific illnesses for which moxa is contraindicated

b) Specific points of the body for which moxa is contraindicated

c) Specific times when moxa is contraindicated

It should also be noted that moxa is inappropriate for a patient who has just eaten or whose stomach is full.

a) Specific illnesses for which moxa is contraindicated

- Bile-related fever[35]
- Blood disorders[36]
- Illnesses caused by fever or a hot condition

b) Specific points on the body for which moxa is contraindicated

- On the doors of the senses, such as the eyes
- On the glands
- On the nerves (veins and arteries), ligaments, and tendons that are not mentioned among the five hundred principal moxa points
- On the urethra (located below the sexual organ) in both men and women
- On the life channel and the procreation channel of the male, found immediately below the sexual organ, to the right and left sides respectively
- On the procreation channel of the female, found immediately below the sexual organ on the right side[37]
- On the optic nerves[38]
- On the tip of the tongue
- On the female genitals

Moxibustion is not appropriate on any of these places, even if the illness is sudden and severe.

c) Specific times when moxa is contraindicated

According to Tibetan medicine, external therapies such as moxibustion, and in particular intense treatments involving the cauterization method, are contraindicated under certain astrological conditions. These factors are explained in detail in Appendix A.[39]

4) Types of Moxa Points

There are two types of moxa points:

a) Localized points related to the illness or pain

b) Points that must be located by the therapist

a) Localized points related to the illness or pain

Localized points include:

- Any painful spot on the body where pressure of the thumb brings relief
- Any spot on the body where strong pressure of the thumb leaves an imprint
- With the exception of all critical nerves and veins, any spot affected by continuous shooting pain in the nerves and veins, and any spot where a problem manifests related to the nerves and veins
- The site of conditions that appear suddenly, such as injuries, cysts, and anthrax, as well as the site of acute swellings

Having clearly identified such localized points in accordance with these categories, one should treat the related conditions using one of the following three methods, whichever is more appropriate:[40]

i) Burning

ii) Heating

iii) Threatening

b) Points that must be located by the therapist

This book is a compilation of the major moxa points specified in the *Last Tantra*[41] along with other points found in the instructions of original medical texts from Shang Shung[42] and Tibet. Altogether, they comprise a total of five hundred highly important, essential, and effective moxa points.

All of these points can be subsumed under three categories:

i) Points on the back

ii) Points on the front

iii) Points on the extremities

i) Individually, the points on the back consist of:

- Eighty points along the spine
- Seventy-four points on the lateral back

ii) The points on the front consist of:

- Sixty-five moxa points on the central front of the torso
- Thirty moxa points on the lateral front of the torso

iii) The points on the extremities consist of:

- Eighty-one points on the head
- Eighty-four points on the arms
- Eighty-six points on the legs

5) HOW TO LOCATE MOXA POINTS

A system of measurement assists in the process of correctly identifying the location of the individual moxa points. This system includes a number of basic units of measurement:

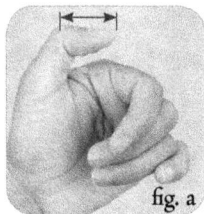
fig. a

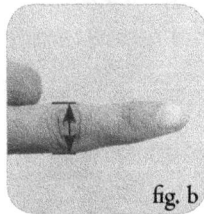
fig. b

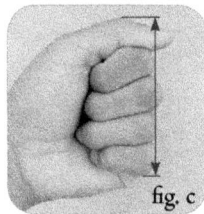
fig. c

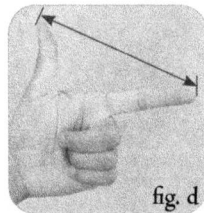
fig. d

- A **thumb** (*tshön* [*mtshon*]), fig. a, refers to the distance from the first phalanx of the thumb to the tip of the thumbnail
- A **finger** (*sor*), fig. b, refers to the width of the second phalanx of the index finger
- A **half finger** (*phun*) is half the width of a finger
- **Four fingers** or **two thumbs** (*chag*) refers to four fingers or two thumbs
- A **fist** (*khyi* [*'khyid*]), fig. c, is equivalent to five fingers and refers to the distance spanned from the thumb to the joint of the little finger when the hand is held in a fist with the thumb on the first phalanx of the index finger
- A **thumb-index span** (*tho* [*mtho*]), fig. d, refers to the distance between the thumb and index finger when stretched apart
- A **scalpel** (*thur*)[43] refers to a unit equal to the length of the instrument for bloodletting, and is equivalent to three thumbs or six fingers

It is important to note that these units of measure are based on the proportion of the patient's hand. The exact location of the moxa points can be accurately determined by marking the patient's proportions on a scalpel or a string and using it as an instrument of measurement.

6) METHODS OF APPLYING MOXA

There are four different methods for applying moxa: cauterizing, burning, heating, and threatening.[44]

a) The Method of Cauterizing

For some types of serious illnesses, such as cysts and tumors, the moxa cone should be placed directly on the actual point. The moxa application must be repeated several times in succession with one cone after the other so as to cauterize the skin. This method is known as cauterizing.[45]

b) The Method of Burning

For Pale Phlegm illnesses,[46] lymphatic disorders, and depressive syndrome,[47] moxa cones should be placed directly on the point many times so as to burn the skin.[48] This method is known as burning.

If one uses the indirect method, for instance by using the small moxa cones produced in Japan, even the burning therapy will not involve problems such as those that can occur when the therapy is performed on a regular basis.[49]

c) The Method of Heating

For severe cases of Wind disorders, illnesses caused by microorganisms such as parasites, obstruction of nerves and blood vessels caused by liquids,[50] and so forth, moxa is more effective if the cone is placed directly on the point five or more times. If the illness is not serious, the point should simply be warmed deeply seven or more times, using heat from the moxa cones. This form of moxa therapy is known as heating.

d) The Method of Threatening

Regardless of the type of illness, when performing moxa on children, the elderly, and pregnant women, the heat from the moxa should be applied to a degree sufficient only to generate a fear of the heat or the feeling of being threatened by the heat. This kind of application is repeated as appropriate, without placing the source of heat directly on the point.[51] This method is known as threatening.

For less severe forms of illnesses of the type that are otherwise indicated for cauterization or burning therapy, practical experience has shown that both the heating and threatening methods can be applied repeatedly with great effect.

7) POST-TREATMENT GUIDELINES

Following those types of moxa requiring direct cauterization or burning, the thumb should be firmly pressed on the spot where the moxa cone was placed.[52] The patient should then immediately stand up and take a few steps. This helps bring the condition of the body back to normal.

Directly after any type of moxa treatment, the patient should refrain from drinking any liquid at all, and that night should take care not to drink cold liquids, including cold water.[53] Moreover, it is very important that for seven days the patient avoid the consumption of acidic foods or drinks (such as spoiled food or fermented products like yogurt, buttermilk, beer, and alcohol), exposure to cold, perspiring as a result of strenuous activities, and sleeping during the daytime.[54]

8) BENEFITS OF MOXA

Successful treatment with moxa has many benefits:

- Clears obstructions within nerves and blood vessels
- Relieves pain related to illnesses
- Alleviates Wind disorders that affect various parts of the body
- Improves poor digestion
- Cures illnesses such as epigastric disorders and tumors
- Potentially arrests the development of cysts and noxious flesh growths, heals chronic wounds
- Reduces swellings of various kinds
- Removes and dries up lymph
- Protects the functioning of the solid and hollow organs
- Increases bodily heat
- Induces mental clarity

In brief, a wide variety of illnesses that are difficult to treat with other therapies can be cured with moxa.

KEY TO MEDICAL SOURCES CITED IN THIS MANUAL

This brief manual of moxibustion uses the following system to indicate the medical sources for the individual points:[55]

A indicates that the point is referred to in *The Last Tantra* (*Phyi ma'i rgyud*), the fourth of the well-known Tibetan medical texts called *The Four Medical Tantras* (*rGyud bzhi*).[56]

B indicates that the point is referred to in *The Moon King* (*Zla ba'i rgyal po*), a famous medical text translated from Sanskrit into Tibetan.[57]

C indicates that the point is referred to in the version of *The Moon King* that was first translated from Sanskrit into Chinese and then from Chinese into Tibetan, referred to here as *Somaraja*.[58]

D indicates that the point is referred to in two medical books on moxa found among the ancient manuscripts from Tun-Huang.[59]

E indicates that the point is referred to in *The White Crystal Mirror: An Extensive Instruction Manual on Moxa* (*Me btsa'i gdams pa rgyas spros shel dkar me long*) by the renowned seventeenth-century doctor Dilmar Geshe Tenzin Phuntshog.[60]

F indicates that the point is referred to in *The Continuous Rainfall of Nectar That Preserves the Life of Beings* (*'Gro ba'i srog 'dzin bdud rtsi'i char rgyun*), a hidden treasure discovered by my root master, the incomparable knowledge holder Changchub Dorje. This extraordinary medical treatise offers methods for curing illnesses of our era.[61]

G indicates that the point is referred to in *The Excellent Wish-Fulfilling Tree: An Indispensable Ornament of the Quintessence of Myriad Treatises on the Art of Healing* (*Tshe rig rgyud 'bum bye ba'i yang bcud zur rgyan nyer mkho dpag bsam ljon shing bzang po*) written by the Shang Shung doctor Khyungchen Pungri Khyungtrul Jigme Namkhai Dorje Yungdrung Gyaltsan.[62]

A   *The Last Tantra*
B   *The Moon King*
C   *Somaraja*
D   Tun-Huang Manuscripts
E   *The White Crystal Mirror*
F   *The Continuous Rainfall of Nectar*
G   *The Excellent Wish-Fulfilling Tree*

PART TWO
Compendium of Points
and Indications

STRUCTURAL OUTLINE

The most important moxa points on the body can be classified into three principal groups, which can be further divided into seven subcategories. In this book, I have presented five hundred of the most important moxa points for a wide variety of different indications:

> POINTS ON THE BACK
>   I: Eighty points along the spine
>   II: Seventy-four points on the lateral back
>
> POINTS ON THE FRONT
>   III: Sixty-five points on the central front of the torso
>   IV: Thirty points on the lateral front of the torso
>
> POINTS ON THE EXTREMITIES (HEAD, ARMS, AND LEGS)[1]
>   V: Eighty-one points on the head
>   VI: Eighty-four points on the arms
>   VII: Eighty-six points on the legs

For each point, I have listed the effects and benefits of applying whichever form of moxa (cauterizing, burning, heating, or threatening) is appropriate, keeping in mind the practitioner's level of skill. Drawings have been provided to clearly show the location of the points.

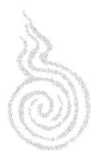

Points on the Back

I. Points Along the Spine

There are eighty very important moxa points along the spine.[2] These points are listed and described below.

Wind Points
I.1-3 ཀྲུང་གསང་ད།

LOCATION | One central point and two lateral points. Apply the appropriate form of moxa (cauterizing, burning, heating, or threatening) on the first vertebra, the equivalent of the seventh cervical vertebra in the Western system. This vertebra, the first of the bones of the spinal column known as *an stong* in Tibetan, protrudes at the nape of the neck when the patient's head is bent forward.[3] If the illness is serious, also include the points located one thumb directly to the right and directly to the left of the central point, using the size of the patient's thumb for measurement.[4]

INDICATIONS |
- Insanity caused by Wind disorders[5] affecting the coronaries[6]
- Confusion
- Trembling
- Loss of speech as a result of Wind disorders
- Arrhythmia
- Sleepiness during the day
- Insomnia
- Loss of hearing

- Headache
- Pale tongue[7]
- Stiffness of the neck
- Bone pain related to chronic fever[8]
- Shortness of breath
- Excessive perspiration
- Back pain[9]
- Loss of appetite
- Head problems caused by lymphatic disorders
- Obstruction of the esophagus caused by Phlegm[10] disorders
- Promotion of well-being in the elderly

SOURCES | A, B, D, F, G

COLD BILE POINTS[11]
1.4-6 གྲང་མཁྲིས་གསང༌།

LOCATION | One central point and two lateral points. Apply the appropriate form of moxa on the second vertebra according to the Tibetan method of counting, the first of the twelve thoracic vertebrae in the Western system. If the illness is serious, include the points located one thumb to the right and left of the central point.

INDICATIONS |
- Bile disorders in general, in particular yellow eyes and yellow complexion related to cold Bile disorder[12]
- Poor digestion
- Heaviness of the upper back
- High blood pressure related to Bile disorders or fever
- Fever that persists internally
- Goiter[13]
- Shortness of breath
- Excessive perspiration
- Back pain
- Bile flowing into the vascular system
- Bile spreading or diffusing into the vascular system
- Extravasation of bile
- Cold Bile disorders
- Loss of appetite
- Wind disorders

SOURCES | A, B, C, D, F, G

GENERAL PHLEGM POINTS
I.7-9 བད་ཀན་སྤྱི་གནས།

LOCATION | One central point and two lateral points. Apply the appropriate form of moxa on the third vertebra (T2). If the illness is serious, include the points located one thumb to the right and left of the central point.

INDICATIONS | *Applied to the central point:*
- Illnesses related to Wind humor of a cold nature[14]
- Bone pain related to chronic fever
- Congestion of blood in the upper back
- Illnesses of the tongue and of the throat
- Illnesses of Pale and Brown Phlegm[15]
- Tumors (Phlegm-related)
- Goiter[16]
- Increase of Phlegm in the upper body, such as the lungs, heart, head, etc.

Applied to all three points:
- Fever that persists internally
- Shortness of breath
- Poor sleep
- Upper back pain and tightness
- Unhappiness
- Nasal congestion
- Dry tongue
- Loss of appetite
- Contagious diseases[17]
- Wind disorders
- Increase of Phlegm

SOURCES | A, B, C, E, F, G

POSTERIOR LUNG LOBE POINTS[18]
I.10-12 གློ་མའི་གནས།

LOCATION | One central point and two lateral points. Apply the appropriate form of moxa on the fourth vertebra (T3). If the illness is serious, include the points located one thumb to the right and left of the central point.

INDICATIONS	*Applied to the central point:*

* Nasal congestion
* Dry mouth and tongue
* Back pain and upper back pain
* Cough with expectoration of hard mucus
* Lacrimation
* Pulmonary diseases related to Wind or Phlegm

Applied to all three points:

* Loss of taste
* Upper back pain caused by pulmonary diseases
* Chronic fever
* Pain and fatigue
* Excessive heat in the body

SOURCES | A, B, C

ANTERIOR LUNG LOBE POINTS[19]
I.13-15 ཨློ་བུའི་གསང་།

LOCATION | One central point and two lateral points. Apply the appropriate form of moxa on the fifth vertebra (T4). If the illness is serious, include the points located one thumb to the right and left of the central point.

INDICATIONS |
* Head problems caused by combined Phlegm and Wind disorders[20]
* Expectoration of blood
* Expectoration of pus
* Continuous cough
* Insanity
* Seizures
* Back pain
* Nausea
* Vomiting
* Trembling of the limbs
* Virulent contagious diseases[21]
* Pulmonary diseases

SOURCES | A, B, C, D, E, F, G

CORONARY POINTS
I.16-18 ཕོག་ཙུའི་རྒྱབ་གསང་།

LOCATION | One central point and two lateral points. Apply the appropriate form of moxa on the sixth vertebra (T5). If the illness is serious, include the points located one thumb to the right and left of the central point.

INDICATIONS |
- Acute pain as if the chest were splitting apart (due to Wind affecting the coronaries)[22]
- Emotional instability[23]
- Insanity
- Trembling
- Fainting and confused state
- Sensation of heaviness
- Cardiac illnesses
- Extreme forgetfulness
- Fainting or seizures
- Outbreaks of pustules or pimples
- Tasting food as unpleasant
- Tightness in the upper back
- Heaviness of the head
- Pericardial effusion
- Emotional upset
- Insomnia
- Irascibility
- Cold sensation in the abdomen, accompanied by poor digestion
- Increase of Phlegm

SOURCES | A, B, C, D, E, F, G

HEART POINTS
I.19-21 སྙིང་གསང་།

LOCATION | One central point and two lateral points. Apply the appropriate form of moxa on the seventh vertebra (T6). If the illness is serious, include the points located one thumb to the right and left of the central point.

INDICATIONS |
- Surging pain in the diaphragm caused by Phlegm
- Sensation of heaviness

* Emotional instability
* Trembling
* Insanity and seizures
* Cardiac illnesses
* Forgetfulness
* Pain and constriction when exposed to cold
* Pain in the floating ribs
* Breathing discomfort
* Insomnia
* Coronary disorders[24]
* Irascibility
* Heaviness of the head
* Emotional upset
* Belching and reflux
* Liver tumors
* Pain or malaise from drinking certain types of water

SOURCES | A, B, C, D, F, G

DIAPHRAGM POINTS
I.22-24   མཆིན་རྡི་བི་གསང་ད།

LOCATION | One central point and two lateral points. Apply the appropriate form of moxa on the eighth vertebra (T7). If the illness is serious, include the points located one thumb to the right and left of the central point.

INDICATIONS |
* Belching and reflux
* Pain in the floating ribs
* Sensation of inner constraint
* Diaphragm problems caused by Phlegm
* Surging pain in the diaphragm
* Pain or malaise when exposed to cold
* Liver tumors
* Liver problems caused by combined Phlegm and Wind disorders
* Acute pain related to blood circulation
* Vomiting of blood caused by liver illnesses
* Impure blood entering into the hollow organs
* Poor assimilation of nutritional essence

* Problems in the liver region

SOURCES | A, B, C, D, E, F, G

LIVER POINTS
I.25-27   མཆིན་པའི་གསང་།

LOCATI ON | One central point and two lateral points. Apply the appropriate form of moxa on the ninth vertebra (T8). If the illness is serious, include the points located one thumb to the right and left of the central point.

INDICATIONS |
* Liver-related pain or malaise caused by combined Phlegm and Wind disorders[25]
* Belching and reflux
* Surging pain in the diaphragm
* Pain or malaise when exposed to cold
* Vomiting of blood caused by liver illnesses
* Throbbing liver
* Reflux of sour or hot liquid
* Retching
* Loss of appetite
* Abdominal distension and pain
* Blood tumors (early stage)
* Liver tumors
* Liver tumors (early stage)
* Internal swellings
* Loss of blood in the semen
* Pain caused by Wind disorders
* Irascibility
* Liver problems caused by Wind humor of a cold nature
* Weak liver[26]

SOURCES | A, B, C, E, F, G

GALLBLADDER POINTS
I.28-30   མཁྲིས་གསང་།

LOCATION | One central point and two lateral points. Apply the appropriate form of moxa on the tenth vertebra (T9). If the illness is serious, include the points located one thumb to the right and left of the central point.

INDICATIONS
- Gallstones
- Tiredness, low energy, sensation of heaviness
- Indigestion
- Yellow eyes
- Yellow complexion
- Constipation
- Sensation of heaviness
- Dark (unhealthy) complexion
- Unclear vision
- Nasal and oral discharge
- Bile in the hollow organs
- Vomiting bile
- Loss of appetite
- Loss of physical radiance
- Lack of digestive heat
- Constant headaches
- Decrease of metabolic heat

SOURCES   A, B, C, E, F, G

SPLEEN POINTS
I.31-33   མཆེར་གསང་།

LOCATION
One central point and two lateral points. Apply the appropriate form of moxa on the eleventh vertebra (T10). If the illness is serious, include the points located one thumb to the right and left of the central point.

INDICATIONS
- Pain in the spleen[27]
- Poor digestion
- Facial emaciation[28]
- Tiredness, low energy, sensation of heaviness
- Heavy sleep
- Excessive belching
- Frequent abdominal distension and sensation of fullness
- Abdominal noises and rumbling

SOURCES   A, B, C, E, F, G

STOMACH POINTS
I.34-36 ཕོ་བའི་གསང་།

LOCATION	One central point and two lateral points. Apply the appropriate form of moxa on the twelfth vertebra (T11). If the illness is serious, include the points located a thumb to the right and left of the central point.
INDICATIONS	• Decrease of digestive heat • Poor digestion • Vomiting • Chronic diarrhea • Epigastric disorders[29] • Chronic gastritis[30] • Illnesses related to Brown Phlegm[31] • Stomach tumors of a cold nature • Stiffness of the lumbar region • Pain in the occipital cavity • Pain in the bones around the eyes
SOURCES	A, B, C, E, F, G

SEMINAL VESICLE AND OVARY POINTS[32]
I.37-39 བསམ་སེའུ་གསང་།

LOCATION	One central point and two lateral points. Apply the appropriate form of moxa on the thirteenth vertebra (T12). If the illness is serious, include the points located one thumb to the right and left of the central point.
INDICATIONS	*Applied to the central point:* • Loss of semen • Heavy menstruation • Discharge of pus and other secretions from the genitals • Emotional instability caused by gynecological disorders • Tumors of the uterus • Increase of Wind humor of a cold nature • Distension and fullness of the lower intestines • Dry stools • Poor digestion • Diarrhea from exposure to sudden temperature changes

- Pain in the five solid organs, including the heart
- Tumors of the large intestine
- Tumors of the small intestine
- Viral or bacterial illnesses

Applied to all three points:

- Promotion of weight loss and physical lightness
- Preservation of vital essence

SOURCES | A, B, C, D, E, F, G

KIDNEY POINTS
I.40-42   མ་ཁལ་གསང་།

LOCATION | One central point and two lateral points. Apply the appropriate form of moxa on the first of the five lumbar vertebrae, the fourteenth vertebra from the central Wind Point. If the illness is serious, include the points located one thumb to the right and left of the central point.

INDICATIONS |
- Kidneys affected by Wind and cold conditions
- Cold sensation and deep chill in the lumbar region
- Colic[33]
- Pain in the large and small intestines
- Urine retention[34]
- Swelling of the genitals
- Impotence
- Constipation and sensation of heaviness
- Semen mixed with white discharge
- Bowel incontinence
- Loss of semen
- Frequent urination
- Burning sensation at tip of the urethra
- Inability to conceive male children
- Kidney disorders of a cold nature

SOURCES | A, B, C, E, F, G

GENERAL SOLID AND HOLLOW ORGAN POINT
I.43   དོན་སྙོད་སྤྱི་གསང་།

LOCATION | One point. Apply moxa on the second lumbar vertebra, the fifteenth vertebra from the central Wind Point. In this case, even if the illness is serious, moxa cannot be applied on the two points to the right and to the left, because these points coincide with the kidneys and with the junction of the anterior and posterior pro-creation channel.[35]

INDICATIONS

- Jaundice
- Increase of Wind humor of a cold nature in the womb
- Infertility
- Aching in the lower part of the small intestine
- Illnesses of the lower body, from the navel down

SOURCES A, B, C, E, F, G

LARGE INTESTINE POINTS
I.44-46 ལོང་གསང་།

LOCATION One central point and two lateral points. Apply the appropriate form of moxa on the third lumbar vertebra, the sixteenth verte-bra from the central Wind Point. If the illness is serious, include the points located one thumb to the right and left of the central point.

INDICATIONS

- Abdominal distension and rumbling in the small and large intes-tines
- Lumbar aches and pains when standing up
- Inability to digest food and drink
- Tumors of the large intestine
- Constipation or diarrhea
- Menstrual problems[36]
- Burning sensation at the tip of the urethra
- Hemorrhoids
- Involuntary release of intestinal gas
- Tumors and other illnesses of the urinary bladder
- Illnesses related to the malfunction of downward-clearing Wind

SOURCES A, B, C, D, E, F, G

SMALL INTESTINE POINTS
I.47-49 རྒྱུ་མའི་གསང་།

LOCATION One central point and two lateral points. Apply the appropriate form of moxa on the fourth lumbar vertebra, the seventeenth vertebra from the central Wind Point. If the illness is serious, include the points located one thumb to the right and left of the central point.

INDICATIONS
- Tumors of the small intestine
- Shortness of breath
- Wind humor of a cold nature
- Chronic fever
- Abdominal distension and empty rumblings when exposed to cold
- Urine retention
- Diarrhea with mucus[37]

SOURCES | A, B, E, F, G

BLADDER POINTS
I.50-52 ལྷུང་པའི་གསང་།

LOCATION | One central point and two lateral points. Apply the appropriate form of moxa on the fifth lumbar vertebra, the eighteenth vertebra from the central Wind Point. If the illness is serious, include the points located one thumb to the right and left of the central point.

INDICATIONS
- Bladder stones
- Urine retention or frequent urination when exposed to cold
- Priapism or swelling of the penis
- Accumulation or discharge of vaginal fluids
- Wind disorders after childbirth
- Swellings in general
- Cold sensation in the knees
- Constipation and urine retention
- Cold sensation in the genitals

SOURCES | A, B, E, F, G

REPRODUCTIVE FLUID POINTS
I.53-55 ཁུ་བའི་གསང་།

LOCATION | One central point and two lateral points. Apply the appropriate form of moxa on the first of the four sacral vertebrae, the nineteenth vertebra from the central Wind Point. If the illness is serious, include the points located one thumb to the right and left of the central point.

INDICATIONS
* Loss of pink semen
* Aching in the bladder[38] and lumbar region
* Dry stools
* Shortness of breath
* Urine retention or frequent urination due to exposure to cold
* Swelling of the limbs
* Drooping of the lower lip
* Stiffness of the muscles of the lumbar region and lower abdomen
* Stiffness and lameness of the muscles in the lower body
* Poor digestion
* Accumulation of lymph
* Leg problems causing difficulties when walking, sitting, and stretching or bending the legs
* Inability to bend the body backward and forward
* Bloody, frothy, or slimy diarrhea
* Loss of semen
* Risk of miscarriage

SOURCES   A, B, D, E, F, G

DOWNWARD-CLEARING WIND POINTS[39]
I.56-58   ཕྱུར་སེལ་གསང༌།

LOCATION   One central point and two lateral points. Apply the appropriate form of moxa on the second sacral vertebra, the twentieth vertebra from the central Wind Point. If the illness is serious, include the points located one thumb to the right and left of the central point.

INDICATIONS
* Genital bleeding
* Diarrhea with bluish slime
* Frequent urination
* Premature ejaculation
* Burning sensation at the tip of the urethra
* Constipation
* Passing of intestinal gas

- Aching or swelling of the testicles
- Aching or swelling at the opening of the vagina
- Aching below the lumbar region when exposed to cold
- Dry stools

SOURCES | A, B, E, F, G

ANUS POINTS
I.59-61　　གཞང་གསང་ད།

LOCATION | One central point and two lateral points. Apply the appropriate form of moxa on the third sacral vertebra, the twenty-first vertebra from the central Wind Point. If the illness is serious, include the points located one thumb to the right and left of the central point.

INDICATIONS |
- Hemorrhoids
- Diarrhea with white and brown mucus
- Shortness of breath
- Surging pain in the lumbar region
- Continuous flashing pain in the hip joints when exposed to cold
- Pain in the anus as if it were splitting
- Diseases of the anus
- Spread and aggravation of Wind humor of a cold nature
- Loss of speech due to Wind disorders or intestinal problems

SOURCES | B, C, E, F, G

GENERAL COLD CONDITION POINTS
I.62-64　　གྲང་བའི་སྐྱི་གསང་ད།

LOCATION | One central point and two lateral points. Apply the appropriate form of moxa on the fourth sacral bone, the protruding bone above the coccyx. If the illness is serious, include the points located one thumb to the right and left of the central point.

INDICATIONS |
- Pain in the hip joints
- Wind humor of a cold nature
- Frequent urination
- Heavy menstruation
- Severe illnesses related to Wind disorders
- Chronic fever

SOURCES | B, C, E, F, G

Tailbone Point
I.65 ཏྲ་མིག་མཇུག་གསང་།

LOCATION | One point. Apply the appropriate form of moxa on the point located on the end of the tailbone.[40]

INDICATIONS
- Blocked lumbar region
- Aching at the anus caused by exposure to cold
- Problems with the lower body caused by Wind disorders affecting the joints
- Diarrhea
- Delirious speech

SOURCES | B, C, D, E, F, G

Nerve Points
I.66-68 རྩ་དཀར་གསང་།

LOCATION | One central point and two lateral points. Apply the appropriate form of moxa on the point located two fingers above the first vertebra (central Wind Point) and the two points located three fingers to the right and left of the central point, avoiding the two tendons or ligaments of the neck.

INDICATIONS
- Ear problems (Wind-related)
- Swelling of the mouth, lips, or face
- Nasal congestion caused by viruses or bacteria associated with Wind disorders
- Toothache related to caries
- Discomfort of the head and neck caused by nerve problems
- Migraine caused by Wind disorders
- Viral or bacterial illnesses of the head[41]

SOURCE: | F

Blood Vessel Points
I.69-71 རྩ་ནག་གསང་།

LOCATION | One central point and two lateral points. Apply the appropriate form of moxa on the point located two fingers above the central

Nerve Point (four fingers above the first vertebra or central Wind Point, coinciding with the center of the three wrinkles found at the nape of the neck) and the two points located three fingers to the right and left of the central point.

INDICATIONS

- Vascular conditions (Wind-related)
- Sensation as if the nerves, skin, and flesh were separating
- Accumulation of lymph (Wind-related)
- Dazed feeling (related to a combination of Blood and Wind)[42]
- Ringing in the ears (related to a combination of Phlegm and Wind)
- Discomfort at the nape of the neck
- Eyesight impairment (Phlegm-related)
- Redness of the eyes (related to a combination of Blood and Wind)
- Combined Blood and Bile disorders
- Conjunctivitis
- Nosebleed

SOURCE | F

VIRUS AND BACTERIA POINTS
I.72-74 སྙིན་གསང་།

LOCATION

One central point and two lateral points. Apply the appropriate form of moxa on the point located two fingers above the central Blood Vessel Point and the two points located three fingers to the right and left of the central point.

INDICATIONS

- Teeth grinding
- Loss of hearing
- Combined Blood and Wind disorders
- Toothache related to caries
- Neurological problems related to contamination[43]
- Rigidity of the nape of the neck as a result of infectious or contagious diseases[44]
- Trauma caused by blows or knocks
- Trauma from serious falls
- Impairment of the mental functions and loss of speech

SOURCE | F

KALO POINTS[45]
I.75-77   ཀ་ལོའི་གསང་།

LOCATION	One central point and two lateral points. Apply the appropriate form of moxa on the point located two fingers above the central Virus and Bacteria Point and the two points located three fingers to the right and left of the central point.
INDICATIONS	• Neurological problems related to contamination or provocations[46] • Fainting • Seizures • Provocations from above[47] • Sudden pain of unidentified origin
SOURCE	F

YAMA POINTS[48]
I.78-80   ཡ་མའི་གསང་།

LOCATION	One central point and two lateral points. Apply the appropriate form of moxa on the point located two fingers above the central Kalo Point and the two points located two fingers to the right and left of the central point.
INDICATIONS	• Combined Wind and Bile disorders • Viral or bacterial illnesses of the blood • Illnesses caused by white and black bacteria or viruses
SOURCE	F

These constitute the eighty most important moxa points along the spine.

II. POINTS ON THE LATERAL BACK

There are seventy-four major moxa points on the lateral parts of the back that are particularly effective. These points are listed and described below.

GATE OF THE SKY POINTS
II.1-10
(81-90) གནས་སྐྱེའི་གསང་།

LOCATION | Two groups of five points. Apply the appropriate form of moxa on the two clusters of five points on the right and left shoulders called the Gate of the Sky.[49] The central point of each cluster is located two fingers from the right and left Wind Point, at the same level as the center of the right and left shoulders. Finger pressure on the central points reveals the ending point of heart-related pain. It is especially important to apply moxa on whichever points in each cluster where there is pain associated with the illness.

From the words of my sacred master, I learned that the central point of each five-point cluster[50] is two fingers away from the right and left Wind Point, and the other points are in the form of a diagonal cross in which each lateral point is one finger from the center. He also said that the two last lateral points of each five-point cluster coincide with the two first lateral points of the clusters referred to below.

INDICATIONS | • Nine types of obstructions of the esophagus related to Phlegm[51]

SOURCE | F

GATE OF THE WIND POINTS[52]
II.11-20
(91-100) རླུང་སྒོའི་གསང་།

LOCATION | Two groups of five points. Apply the appropriate form of moxa on the five-point clusters as described above, where the central point is located two fingers to the right and left of the central Gate of the Sky Point.

INDICATIONS | • Acute pain at the meeting point of the heart and coronaries[53]

SOURCE | F

GATE OF CONTAMINATION POINTS[54]
II.21-30 གྲིབ་སྒོའི་གསང་།
(101-110)

LOCATION	Two groups of five points. Apply the appropriate form of moxa on the five-point clusters as described above, where the central point is located two fingers to the right and left of the central Gate of the Wind Point.
INDICATIONS	• Illnesses resulting from harmful effects of provocations[55]
SOURCE	F

CENTRAL SHOULDER POINTS[56]
II.31-40 ཕྲག་མིག་གི་གསང་།
(111-120)

LOCATION	Two groups of five points. Apply the appropriate form of moxa on the five-point clusters as described above, where the central point is located two fingers to the right and left of the central Gate of Contamination Point, that is, on the two central points on the shoulders.[57]
INDICATIONS	• Neurological and vascular conditions caused by contamination • Persistent, low-grade fever
SOURCE	F

SHOULDER REGION POINTS
II.41-48 ཕྲག་འཁོར་གསང་།
(121-128)

LOCATION	Two groups of four points. Apply the appropriate form of moxa on the four points located on the four sides of the clusters centered around the points two fingers from the right and left Central Shoulder Point.[58]
INDICATIONS	• Combined Blood and Wind disorders caused by the five types of Wind[59] • Conditions related to contamination • Conditions related to provocations • Problems in the inner and outer parts of the body caused by minor Wind disorders or scattered Wind • Diseases contracted from wild animals[60]

SOURCE | F

NERVE WIND POINTS

II.49-50 ཙ་དགར་རྫུར་གསང་།
(129-130)

LOCATION | One point on each side. Apply the appropriate form of moxa on the points located four thumbs from each lateral Wind Point (I.2 and I.3), parallel to the line of the shoulder, and then three and a half fingers down. [61]

INDICATIONS | • Nerve-related numbness
• Nerve pain

SOURCE | E

LATERAL MINOR TENDON POINTS

II.51-52 འཆུ་ཕྱན་ཟྲར་གསང་།
(131-132)

LOCATION | One point on each side. Apply the appropriate form of moxa on the points located one thumb from each Nerve Wind Point toward the center of the back and half a finger down from there.

INDICATIONS | • Lameness related to the nerves
• Loss of muscular control due to neurological problems
• Neurological problems on certain days of the lunar calendar[62]

SOURCE | E

SHEEP TAIL POINTS

II.53-54 ལུག་མཇུག་གསང་།
(133-134)

LOCATION | One point on each side. Apply the appropriate form of moxa on the points located one thumb below each Nerve Wind Point.

INDICATIONS | • Pus formation in the lungs

SOURCE | E

LATERAL LUNG CAVITY POINTS[63]

II.55-56 གློ་ཕུག་ཟྲར་གསང་།
(135-136)

LOCATION | One point on each side. Apply the appropriate form of moxa on the points located two thumbs, or four fingers, directly to the right and left of the fourth vertebra (T3).[64]

INDICATIONS	• Spread of pus related to chronic pulmonary diseases
SOURCE	E

CENTER OF THE MIRROR POINTS
II.57-58
(137-138)   མེ་ལོང་དཀྱིལ་གསང་།

LOCATION	One point on each side. Apply the appropriate form of moxa on the points located one fist, or five fingers, below the central ridge of each shoulder blade.[65]
INDICATIONS	• Spread of pus in the lungs • Consumptive pulmonary diseases (such as tuberculosis) • Pulmonary collapse • Bluish complexion • Nerve problems (Wind-related)
SOURCES	E, F, G

HEART/CORONARY POINTS
II.59-60
(139-140)   སྙིང་རྩོག་གསང་།

LOCATION	One point on each side. Apply the appropriate form of moxa on the points located two fingers below the right and left Center of the Mirror Point.
INDICATIONS	• Pain at the meeting point of the heart and coronaries[66] • Malfunction of the lungs • Conditions related to contamination or provocations • Insanity[67]
SOURCE	F

UPPER LUNG POINTS
II.61-62
(141-142)   གློ་སྟེང་གསང་།

LOCATION	One point on each side. Apply the appropriate form of moxa on the points located two thumbs below the right and left Center of the Mirror Point.

INDICATIONS	• Coughing • Vomiting • Pus formation in the lungs
SOURCES	E, F

STOMACH TUMOR POINTS
II.63-64
(143-144)   ཕོ་བའི་སྐྲན་གསང་།

LOCATION	One point on each side. Apply the appropriate form of moxa on the points located two fingers below the right and left Upper Lung Point.
INDICATIONS	• Stomach disorders (Wind-related)[68] • Indigestion • Stomach cancer • Viral or bacterial illnesses • Wind disorders arising after a fever • Chronic gastritis[69]
SOURCE	F

UPPER PULMONARY RIB POINTS
II.65-66
(145-146)   གློ་སྲང་རྩིབས་གསང་།

LOCATION	One point on each side. Apply the appropriate form of moxa on the points located two fingers below the right and left Stomach Tumor Point, on the same line as the Center of the Mirror Point.
INDICATIONS	• Wind or pus affecting the bronchial tubes or the lower lungs • Cancer of the intestine or colon • Aggravation of viral or bacterial illnesses • Toxic condition caused by indigestion • Loss of nutritional essence in the viscera or hollow organs[70]
SOURCES	E, F

PULMONARY RIB POINTS
II.67-68
(147-148)   གློ་བའི་རྩིབས་གསང་།

LOCATION	One point on each side. Apply the appropriate form of moxa on the points located one thumb from the right and left Upper Pul-

monary Rib Point in the direction of the armpits.

INDICATIONS
- Pus formation in the lungs
- Coughing
- Obstructed breathing
- Pulmonary problems associated with Wind disorders[71]
- Problems with the ribs

SOURCE E

LATERAL LIVER POINT
II.69
(149) ཨ་ཚེན་པའི་ཟུར་གསང་།

LOCATION One point. Apply the appropriate form of moxa on the point located two thumbs to the right of the ninth vertebra (T8).[72]

INDICATIONS
- Pain in the liver
- Liver tumors
- Liver illnesses

SOURCE E

LATERAL SPLEEN POINT
II.70
(150) ཨ་ཚེར་པའི་ཟུར་གསང་།

LOCATION One point. Apply the appropriate form of moxa on the point located two thumbs to the left of the ninth vertebra (T8).

INDICATIONS
- Pain in the spleen
- Spleen tumors
- Illnesses of the spleen

SOURCE E

LUNG AND KIDNEY POINTS
II.71-72
(151-152) གློ་མཁལ་གསང་།

LOCATION One point on each side. Apply the appropriate form of moxa on the point located one thumb below the right and left Upper Pulmonary Rib Point.

INDICATIONS
- Illnesses that present pus formation in the lungs

- Ureteral trauma
- Viral or bacterial kidney disorders
- Kidney disorders (Wind-related)[73]

SOURCES | E, F

URETER POINTS

II.73-74
(153-154)

མ་ཁལ་ཕྲག་གསང་།

LOCATION | One point on each side. Apply the appropriate form of moxa on the points located two thumbs to the right and left of the fourteenth vertebra (LI).[74]

INDICATIONS |
- Viral or bacterial kidney disorders
- Kidney cysts
- Kidney tumors
- Kidney disorders accompanied by blood or pus in the urine

SOURCE | F

These constitute the seventy-four most important and most effective moxa points on the lateral parts of the back.

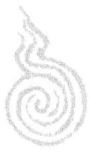

Points on the Front

III. POINTS ON THE CENTRAL FRONT OF THE TORSO

There are sixty-five major moxa points on the central front of the torso that are particularly effective. These points are listed and described below.

POINT ABOVE THE ADAM'S APPLE
III.1
(155) ཨོལ་མདུད་སྟེང་གསབ་ད།

LOCATION	One point. Apply the appropriate form of moxa (burning, heating, or threatening) on the point located four fingers up from the base of the neck or two fingers above the Adam's apple.[75]
INDICATIONS	◦ Consumptive pulmonary diseases (such as tuberculosis) ◦ Hoarseness ◦ Continuous nosebleed ◦ Illness or pain affecting the upper back ◦ Phlegm constricting the pharynx and impeding swallowing[76]
SOURCES	D, F

LATERAL POINTS ABOVE THE ADAM'S APPLE
III.2-3
(156-157) ཨོལ་སྟེང་འགྲམ་གསབ་ད།

LOCATION	One point on each side. Apply the appropriate form of moxa on

the points located two fingers to the right and left of the Point Above the Adam's Apple, taking care to avoid the glands.[77]

INDICATIONS
* Problems with the major and minor jugular veins of the neck[78]
* Hoarseness
* Cancer of the blood
* Angina[79] and infectious diseases

SOURCE   F

LATERAL ADAM'S APPLE POINTS
III.4-5
(158-159) ཨོལ་འགྲམ་གསང་།

LOCATION   One point on each side. Apply the appropriate form of moxa on the points located two fingers to the right and left of the Adam's apple.

INDICATIONS
* Phlegm illnesses constricting the esophagus[80]
* Vomiting

SOURCES   E, F

JUGULAR NOTCH POINT
III.6
(160) ཀེ་སྟོང་གསང་།

LOCATION   One point. Apply the appropriate form of moxa in the soft tissue of the jugular notch or *tsa ra khung*, located where the three bone segments in the neck area meet.[81]

INDICATIONS
* Sensation of being lost
* Pericardial effusion
* Hiccups
* Hoarseness[82]
* Goiter[83]
* Stiffness of the neck
* Quavering voice
* Panic attacks
* Constriction of the esophagus and chest accompanied by a choking sensation, caused by an accumulation of Phlegm
* Inability to vomit

* Illnesses caused by an accumulation of Phlegm

SOURCES | A, B, C, F, G

CORONARIES/HEART UNION POINT
III.7
(161) ཕྲོག་སྙིང་འདོམ་གསང་།

LOCATION | One point. Apply the appropriate form of moxa on the point located in the superficial depression where the collarbone and sternum join at the base of the neck.

INDICATIONS | * Stiffness of the neck
* Constriction at the heart
* Hiccups
* Hoarseness
* Goiter (Wind-related)[84]
* Illnesses provoked by Phlegm

SOURCES | A, B, D, E, F, G

EYE OF THE CROW POINTS
III.8-10
(162-164) བྱ་རོག་མིག་གསང་།

LOCATION | One central point and two lateral points. Apply the appropriate form of moxa on the point located one thumb below the Jugular Notch Point and the two points located one thumb to the right and left of the central point.

INDICATIONS | *Applied to all three points:*
* High blood pressure
* Sensation of tightness in the upper back (related to a combination of Blood and Wind)
* Pus formation in the lungs
* Panting
* Coughing when tired or fatigued
* Obstructed breathing
Applied to the lateral points:[85]
* Depressive syndrome[86]
* Emotional upset

SOURCES | B, C, E, F

POINTS BETWEEN THE LUNGS

III.11-13
(165-167)

གློ་བའི་བར་གསང་།

LOCATION

One central point and two lateral points. Apply the appropriate form of moxa on the point located one thumb below the Eye of the Crow Point and the two points located one thumb to the right and left of the central point.

INDICATIONS

- Pulmonary diseases of a hot nature
- Halitosis
- Fever
- Cysts
- Throbbing lungs
- Strong cough with expectoration
- Wind humor affecting the upper body

SOURCES

B, C, E, F

GRAPE POINTS

III.14-16
(168-170)

རྒུན་འབྲུམ་གསང་།

LOCATION

One central point and two lateral points. Apply the appropriate form of moxa on the point located one thumb plus one half finger below the Point Between the Lungs and the two points located one thumb to the right and left of the central point.

INDICATIONS

- Pulmonary diseases of a hot nature
- Halitosis
- Fever
- Cysts
- Throbbing lungs
- Strong cough
- Wind humor affecting the upper body
- Acute cardiac pain radiating from the chest to the back
- Pulmonary diseases of a cold nature

SOURCES

B, C, E, F

MAJOR HEART POINTS

III.17-19
(171-173) སྙིང་གསང་ཆེན་མོ།

LOCATION	One central point and two lateral points. Apply the appropriate form of moxa on the point located one thumb plus one half finger below the Grape Point, at the level of the nipples (known as the "central part of the chest between black and white")[87] and the two points located one thumb to the right and left of the central point.
INDICATIONS	• Arrhythmia • Emotional instability • Unhappiness • Loss of appetite • Inability to keep food down
SOURCES	A, B, C, E, F, G

BREAST POINT

III.20
(174) ནུ་མའི་གསང་།

LOCATION	One point. Apply the appropriate form of moxa on the point located one half finger below the Major Heart Point.
INDICATIONS	• Illnesses of the breast region • Hot breath issuing from the nose and mouth[88] • Lymph spreading to the heart • Indigestion in children accompanied by pain in the chest • Pain in the right and left sides of the torso
SOURCES	B, C, E, F

EPIGASTRIC POINTS[89]

III.21-23
(175-177) ཕྱིན་གསང་།

LOCATION	One central point and two lateral points. Apply the appropriate form of moxa on the point located one half finger below the Breast Point and the two points located one thumb plus one half finger to the right and left of the central point.
INDICATIONS	• Heartburn[90]

* Reflux of sour liquid
* Metallic taste or lack of taste in the mouth accompanied by loss of appetite
* Tightness in the upper back
* Belching
* Hyperventilation
* Indigestion

SOURCES | A, B, C, D, E, F

XIPHOID POINT
III.24
(178) ཕྱིན་ཁྲུམས་གསང་།

LOCATION | One point. Apply the appropriate form of moxa on the point located one thumb above the tip of the xiphoid process.

INDICATIONS |
* Heartburn
* Metallic taste or lack of taste in the mouth
* Reflux of sour liquid
* Belching
* Tightness in the upper back
* Hyperventilation

SOURCE | B, C, E, F

LOWER XIPHOID POINT
III.25
(179) ཕྱིན་ཁྲུམས་འོག་གསང་།

LOCATION | One point. Apply the appropriate form of moxa on the point located one half thumb, or one finger, below the Xiphoid Point.

INDICATIONS |
* Cardiac illnesses
* Depressive syndrome
* Pericardial effusion
* Unhappiness and sighing
* Intercostal pain resulting from minor Wind disorders or scattered Wind

SOURCE | F

XIPHOID TIP POINTS
III.26-28
(180-182)
ཊྭེན་སྤུའི་གསང༌།

LOCATION | One central point and two lateral points. Apply the appropriate form of moxa on the point located at the center of the xiphoid process tip and the two points located one thumb to the right and left of the central point.

INDICATIONS |
- Brown Phlegm disorders manifesting symptoms in the upper body[91]
- Epigastric disorders
- Tightness in the upper back and poor digestion
- Excessive nasal mucus
- Diarrhea
- Vomiting
- Belching
- Reflux of sour liquid
- Abdominal distension
- Metallic taste or lack of taste in the mouth
- Nausea
- Loss of appetite
- Swelling of the face
- Pain in the side of the torso below the liver
- Common cold
- Heaviness at the front of the head
- Breathing problems

SOURCES | B, C, E, F

TUMOR POINTS
III.29-31
(183-185)
སྐྲན་གསང༌།

LOCATION | One central point and two lateral points. Apply the appropriate form of moxa on the point located one thumb below the central Xiphoid Tip Point and the two points located one thumb to the right and left of the central point.

INDICATIONS |
- Frequent reflux of sour liquid
- Pain in the side of the torso below the liver
- Swelling of the face
- Poor digestion

- Diarrhea
- Food poisoning
- Vomiting
- Breathing discomfort
- Passing of intestinal gas
- Belching
- Abdominal distension beginning in the afternoon

Applied to the lateral point on the patient's right side:
- Liver tumors

Applied to the lateral point on the patient's left side:
- Abdominal distension and pain caused by spleen disorders
- Various types of diarrhea

SOURCES | A, B, C, D, E, F, G

FIRE-ACCOMPANYING WIND POINTS

III.32-34
(186-188)   མེ་མཚམས་གསར་།

LOCATION | One central point and two lateral points. Apply the appropriate form of moxa on the point located four thumbs below the central Xiphoid Tip Point and the two points located one thumb to the right and left of the central point.

INDICATIONS |
- Pain in the upper part of the liver
- Migraine (Wind-related)
- Vomiting of blood caused by liver illnesses
- Epigastric tumors (Phlegm-related)
- Tumors related to Brown Phlegm[92]
- Increase of Wind humor of a cold nature
- Abdominal distension
- Swelling of the face
- Pain in the side of the torso below the liver
- Passing of intestinal gas
- Respiratory problems
- Difficult digestion
- Lack of digestive heat[93]

SOURCES | A, B, C, D, E, F, G

NAVEL REGION POINTS
III.35-37
(189-191)
ལྟེ་ཁྱུད་གསང་།

LOCATION	One central point and two lateral points. Apply the appropriate form of moxa on the point located one thumb above the navel and the two points located one thumb to the right and left of the central point.
INDICATIONS	• Urine retention and loss of nutritional essence in women[94] • Fever
SOURCE	D

POINT ABOVE THE NAVEL
III.38
(192)
ལྟེ་གོང་གསང་།

LOCATION	One point. Apply the appropriate form of moxa on the point located one finger above the upper edge of the navel.
INDICATIONS	• Hemorrhages caused by fevers • Pain and weakness caused by cold illnesses • Swelling of the small intestine due to edema[95] • Cold sensation in the feet and in the lower body • Internal swellings and urine retention after childbirth (Wind-related)
SOURCE	D

NAVEL CAVITY POINT
III.39
(193)
ལྟེ་ཁུང་གསང་།

LOCATION	One point. Apply the appropriate form of moxa in the center of the navel.
INDICATIONS	• Internal gynecological disorders in general • Bleeding between menstrual periods • Wind disorders after childbirth • Abdominal distension • Swellings in general • Infertility • Resurgence of toxic condition
SOURCES	B, C, E

DESCENDING COLON POINTS[96]

III.40-41
(194-195)   ཕོང་ཐེར་གསང་།

LOCATION	One point on each side. Apply the appropriate form of moxa on the two points located one thumb to the right and left of the navel.
INDICATIONS	• Tumors of the large intestine • Loss or lack of semen • Bleeding between menstrual periods or absence of menstruation • Bile affecting the small intestine[97] • Infertility • Frequent abdominal distension and rumbling • Resurgence of a toxic condition • Wind humor of a cold nature
SOURCES	A, B, C, D, E, F, G

UPPER SMALL INTESTINE POINTS

III.42-44
(196-198)   རྒྱུ་སྟོད་གསང་།

LOCATION	One central point and two lateral points. Apply the appropriate form of moxa on the point located one thumb below the navel and the two points located one thumb to the right and left of the central point.
INDICATIONS	• Diarrhea caused by Wind humor affecting the small intestine • Pulmonary diseases and diseases of the large intestine • Abdominal noises and rumbling • Reflux of hot liquid • Urine retention • Pain or malaise when exposed to cold • Severe consumptive edema[98]
SOURCES	A, B, C, D, E, F, G

STOMACH AND LARGE INTESTINE POINTS

III.45-47
(199-201)   ཕོ་ལོང་གསང་།

LOCATION	One central point and two lateral points. Apply the appropriate form of moxa on the point located one thumb below the navel

and the two points located five half fingers, or one thumb plus one half finger, to the right and left of the central point.

INDICATIONS ・ Urine retention and related pain and discomfort

SOURCE D

LOWER SMALL INTESTINE POINTS
III.48-50
(202-204) རྒྱུ་སྲད་གསང་།

LOCATION One central point and two lateral points. Apply the appropriate form of moxa on the point located one thumb below the Upper Small Intestine Point and the two points located one thumb to the right and left of the central point.

INDICATIONS
・ Small intestine conditions caused by Wind of a cold nature
・ Uterine pain
・ Problems in the lumbar region
・ Kidney disorders caused by trauma
・ Viral or bacterial infections
・ Diarrhea
・ Swelling of the penis
・ Frequent urination
・ Pain at the tip of the urethra
・ Irregular menstruation
Indications specified in The Continuous Rainfall of Nectar:[99]
・ Malfunction of the bladder
・ Severe edema[100]
・ Uterine illnesses
・ Disorders of the female reproductive system
・ Kidney disorders caused by Brown Phlegm[101]
・ Lymphatic disorders
・ Kidney disorders caused by trauma
・ Swelling of the scrotum
・ Wind humor of a cold nature affecting the lower body
・ Formation of cysts of a cold nature caused by loss of semen or menstrual blood
・ Cysts and tumors
・ Decrease of stomach functions
・ Viral or bacterial infections

° Incurable illnesses caused by poisons of a cold nature[102]

SOURCES | A, B, C, D, E, F, G

FRONT BLADDER POINTS
III.51-53
(205-207)
 སྐྲང་པའི་མཐུན་གསང་།

LOCATION | One central point and two lateral points. Apply the appropriate form of moxa on the point located one thumb below the Lower Small Intestine Point and the two points located one thumb to the right and left of the central point.

INDICATIONS |
° Infertility
° Risk of miscarriage
° Urine retention or frequent urination when exposed to cold
° Disorders of the female reproductive system (Wind-related)
° Diarrhea
° Priapism
° Swelling of the scrotum and penis
° Tightness and pain in the navel region
° Wind disorders after childbirth
° Continuous menstruation
° Recurrent absence of menstruation
° Disorders of the female reproductive system in general

SOURCES | A, B, C, D, E, F, G

SOFT BLADDER POINT[103]
III.54
(208)
སྐྲང་སྟེའི་གསང་།

LOCATION | One point. Apply the appropriate form of moxa on the point located one thumb below the central Front Bladder Point.

INDICATIONS |
° Uterine illnesses
° Disorders of a cold nature of the female reproductive system
° Disorders of a cold nature related to the kidneys and lumbar region
° Pain or malaise from drinking certain types of water
° Problems with the legs or feet

SOURCES | B, C, E, F

LONG CREASE POINTS
III.55-57
(209-211)
གཉེར་རིང་གསང་།

LOCATION | One central point and two lateral points. Apply the appropriate form of moxa on the point located at the center of the long crease[104] and the two points located one thumb to the right and left of the central point.

INDICATIONS |
* Blood disorders
* Lymphatic disorders
* Bile disorders[105]
* Fever associated with a combined disturbance of the three humors
* Pain in the kidneys and lumbar region
* Swelling of the testicles
* Swelling of the female genitals
* Swelling of the head and face
* Viral or bacterial illnesses
* Cysts in the female reproductive system

SOURCES | B, C, E, F

GENITAL REGION POINTS
III.58-60
(212-214)
མྲང་མཚམས་གསང་།

LOCATION | One central point and two lateral points. Apply the appropriate form of moxa on the point located two fingers above the male or female genitals and the two points located one thumb to the right and left of the central point.

INDICATIONS |
* Frothy and slimy diarrhea
* Urine retention
* Swelling in the lower body
* Slow metabolism
* Pink or light-colored menstrual blood
* Vaginal discharge

SOURCES | B, C, D, E, F

FERTILITY POINTS
III.61-62
(215-216)
ཕྱིད་གསང་།

LOCATION	One point on each side. Apply the appropriate form of moxa on the points located in the area of the two arteries to the right and left of the male or female genitals.[106]
INDICATIONS	• Fertility problems • Risk of miscarriage[107]
SOURCES	E, G

PERINEAL POINT
III.63
(217)
ཚིག་གསང་།

LOCATION	One point. Apply the appropriate form of moxa on the point located two fingers from the male or female genitals in the direction of the anus.
INDICATIONS	• Trembling • Insanity • Heaviness of the upper back and heavy breathing • Swelling of the penis • Swelling of the vaginal labia • Loss of semen • Bleeding between menstrual periods or absence of menstruation • Constriction of the blood vessels
SOURCES	B, C, E, F

LATERAL PERINEAL POINTS
III.64-65
(218-219)
རུ་གསང་།

LOCATION	One point on each side. Apply the appropriate form of moxa on the points located one thumb to the right and left of the Perineal Point on male and female patients. The point on the patient's right is called *Mönru* for women and *Sharu* for men. The point on the patient's left for women is called *Sharu* for women and *Mönru* for men.

INDICATIONS | *Applied to both points:*
* Impotence resulting from excessive sexual intercourse
Applied to the Mönru Point (on the left for men and the right for women):
* Urine retention and frequent urination
Applied to the Sharu Point for women (on the left):
* Risk of miscarriage
Applied to the Sharu Point for men (on the right):
* Low fertility

SOURCES | B, C, E, F

These constitute the sixty-four most important and most effective moxa points on the central front of the torso.

IV. POINTS ON THE LATERAL FRONT OF THE TORSO

There are thirty major moxa points on both sides of the front of the torso that are particularly effective. These points are listed and described below.

LATERAL CORONARIES/HEART UNION POINTS

IV.1-2
(220-221) ཤོག་སྟེང་རུར་གསང་།

LOCATION	One point on each side. Apply the appropriate form of moxa (burning, heating, or threatening) on the two points located five fingers to right and left of the point located two fingers up from the Jugular Notch Point.[108] The central point cannot be used for moxa because the air passages are located here.
INDICATIONS	• Obstruction of the life-sustaining Wind[109] • Foggy feeling • Impaired vision[110] • Acute cardiac pain radiating from the chest to the back
SOURCES	A, B, D, E, F

COMBINED BLOOD AND WIND POINTS

IV.3-4
(222-223) ཁྲག་རླུང་གསང་།

LOCATION	One point on each side. Apply the appropriate form of moxa on the two points located five fingers to the right and left of the point located two fingers above the Union of the Coronaries and Heart Point.[111]
INDICATIONS	• Enlargement of the heart and decrease in physical strength (related to a combination of Blood and Wind) • Gasping • Inability to bend forward, backward, or to the sides • Goiter[112] • Formation of tumors related to the four humors[113] • Vomiting • Indigestion
SOURCE	F

COLLARBONE JUNCTION POINTS
IV.5-6
(224-225) ཐོག་མཐོའི་གསང་།

LOCATION	One point on each side. Apply the appropriate form of moxa on the two points located on the prominent curve on the collar-bone[114] on the right and left sides.
INDICATIONS	• Chronic wounds that do not heal • Wounds, ulcers, or cysts that are difficult to heal • Bone pain (Wind-related)
SOURCES	B, C, E, G

VALLEY ABOVE THE COLLARBONE POINTS
IV.7-8
(226-227) ཐོག་གཡོང་གསང་།

LOCATION	One point on each side. Apply the appropriate form of moxa on the point located in the valley above each collarbone.
INDICATIONS	• Dry cough • Chest pain • Pulmonary diseases accompanied by heavy coughing
SOURCES	B, C, E

COUGH POINTS
IV.9-10
(228-229) ཐོ་ལུའི་གསང་།

LOCATION	One point on each side. Apply the appropriate form of moxa on the points of the neck located four fingers above the center of each collarbone.
INDICATIONS	• Coughing blood • Continuous cough • Pulmonary diseases accompanied by heavy coughing
SOURCES	B, C, E, F

BUBRON POINTS[115]
IV.11-12
(230-231) བུབ་རོན་གསང་།

LOCATION	One point on each side. Apply the appropriate form of moxa on

the points located one thumb above the right and left Eye of the Crow Point.[116]

INDICATIONS
• Acute pain extending from the chest to the back (Wind-related)
• Coughing
• Difficulty in moving the arms

SOURCES   D, E

LATERAL EYE OF THE CROW POINTS
IV.13-14
(232-233)   བྱ་མིག་ཟུར་གསང་།

LOCATION
One point on each side. Apply the appropriate form of moxa on the points located one thumb to the right and left of the right and left Eye of the Crow Point.[117]

INDICATIONS
• High blood pressure
• Pulmonary and cardiac complaints
• Coronary disorders (Wind-related)[118]
• Tightness in the upper back
• Gasping
• Excessive yawning
• Nausea
• Dizziness
• Pain at the meeting point of the heart and coronaries[119]

SOURCE   E

UNION OF LUNGS AND HEART POINTS
IV.15-16
(234-235)   གློ་སྙིང་འདོམ་གསང་།

LOCATION
One point on each side. Apply the appropriate form of moxa on the points located one thumb to the right and left of the right and left Major Heart Point.[120]

INDICATIONS
• Nausea
• Vomiting
• Loss of appetite

SOURCES   D, E

POINTS ABOVE THE BREAST
IV.17-18
(236-237) ནུ་གོང་གསང་།

LOCATION	One point on each side. Apply the appropriate form of moxa on the points located three fingers above the nipples of the right and left breasts.
INDICATIONS	• Migraine (Wind-related) • Dark (unhealthy) complexion • Cerebral illnesses or pain
SOURCE	D

LATERAL XIPHOID POINTS
IV.19-20
(238-239) སྙིན་ཁྲམས་ཟུར་གསང་།

LOCATION	One point on each side. Apply the appropriate form of moxa on the points located one finger to the right and left of the point one thumb above the tip of the xiphoid process.
INDICATIONS	• Heartburn (Phlegm-related) • Metallic taste or lack of taste in the mouth • Reflux of sour liquid • Belching • Tightness in the upper back and hyperventilation • Cardiac illnesses • Depressive syndrome • Pericardial effusion • Unhappiness and sighing • Intercostal pain resulting from minor Wind disorders or scattered Wind *Indications specified in* The Continuous Rainfall of Nectar:[121] • Chronic gastritis (Phlegm-related)[122] • Pain in the waist when bending forward or backward • Wind humor of a cold nature • Nausea • Lack of appetite • Deeply entrenched Brown Phlegm[123] • Spreading Brown Phlegm • Chronic fever

* Turbid fever[124]
* Residue of Brown Phlegm after a fever

SOURCES | B, C, E, F

LATERAL LIVER AND SPLEEN POINTS

IV.21-22
(240-241) མཆིན་མཆེར་རུར་གསང་།

LOCATION | One point on each side. Apply the appropriate form of moxa on the two points located on the long (tenth) ribs on the right and left.[125] The left is the point of the spleen, the right the point of the liver.

INDICATIONS |
* Indigestion (various types)
* Diarrhea
* Strong pain (in the liver and spleen)

SOURCES | B, C

LATERAL FIRE-ACCOMPANYING WIND POINTS

IV.23-28
(242-247) མེ་མཉམ་རུར་གསང་།

LOCATION | Three points on each side. Apply the appropriate form of moxa on the two points located three fingers to the right and left of the point located four fingers above the navel and the four points located two fingers above and below these points.

INDICATIONS |
* Indigestion
* Vomiting (Phlegm-related)
* Diarrhea
* Poor digestion
* Food poisoning
* Contagious diseases
* Deeply entrenched Brown Phlegm[126]

SOURCE | F

INNER COLON POINTS

IV.29-30
(248-249) ལོང་ཕུགས་གསང་།

LOCATION | One point on each side. Apply the appropriate form of moxa on the points located one thumb to the right and left of the right and left Descending Colon Point.[127]

INDICATIONS

- Tumors of the large intestine
- Abdominal distension and rumbling
- Inability to walk
- Bile disorders of a cold nature
- Poor digestion caused by Wind humor of a cold nature
- Severe diarrhea

SOURCES

A, B, C, E, F, G

These constitute the thirty most important and most effective moxa points on the lateral front of the torso.

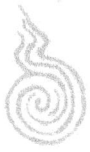

Points on the Extremities

There are two hundred fifty-one major moxa points on the extremities (the head, arms, and legs) that are particularly effective and indispensible.

V. POINTS ON THE HEAD

There are eighty-one particularly beneficial moxa points on the head, the central extremity. These points are listed and described below.

CROWN OF THE HEAD POINT

V.1
(250)   གཙུག་གསང་།

LOCATION	One point. Apply the appropriate form of moxa (golden needle,[128] burning, heating, or threatening) on the crown of the head, which is located at the crossing point of two strings, one extending from the center of the forehead to the center of the occipital bone and one from the tip of the right ear to the tip of the left ear.
INDICATIONS	• Dizziness (Wind-related)[129] • Epilepsy • Dazed feeling • Eyesight impairment caused by Pale Phlegm[130] • Yellow eyes • Yellow complexion • Viral or bacterial illnesses of the brain

- Rigidity of the nape of the neck due to contagious diseases[131]
- Swelling of the face
- Migraine[132]
- Brain tumors
- Minor cerebral illnesses
- Nosebleed

SOURCES | A, B, C, D, E, F, G

LATERAL CROWN OF THE HEAD POINTS
V.2-3
(251-252)   གཙུག་ཟུར་གསང་།

LOCATION | One point on each side. Apply the appropriate form of moxa (burning, heating, or threatening) on the two points located two fingers to the right and left of the Crown of the Head Point in the direction of the tips of the ears.

INDICATIONS
- Otitis[133]
- Cranial pain or pain in the eye sockets
- Pain in the eyeballs (related to a combination of Phlegm and Wind)
- Aggravated and combined Phlegm and Blood disorders
- Concentration or dispersion of viruses or bacteria in the blood
- Combined Phlegm and Blood disorders that spread through the head

SOURCE | F

POINTS BETWEEN THE CROWN AND EARS
V.4-5
(253-254)   རྣ་གཙུག་གསང་།

LOCATION | One point on each side. Apply the appropriate form of moxa on the points located two fingers to the right and left of the right and left Lateral Crown of the Head Point in the direction of the tips of the ears.

INDICATIONS
- Complaints related to the torso, lungs, and upper back
- Depressive syndrome
- Abnormal blood conditions
- Upper back pain
- Goiter[134]

* Loss of voice

SOURCE | F

MIGRAINE POINTS
V.6-7
(255-256) ཀྲུ་ད་གཉེར་གསང་།

LOCATION | One point on each side. Apply the appropriate form of moxa on the points located two fingers towards the forehead from the right and left Point Between the Crown and Ears.

INDICATIONS |
* Migraine[135]
* Dizziness
* Impaired vision[136]

SOURCE | F

NEST OF VIRUS AND BACTERIA POINTS[137]
V.8-9
(257-258) ཉྱིན་ཆོང་གསང་།

LOCATION | One point on each side. Apply the appropriate form of moxa on the points located two fingers towards the front of the head from the right and left Migraine Point.

INDICATIONS |
* Facial paresis
* Moving, shifting, or pulling of the lower jaw
* Nasal congestion
* Rhinitis[138]

SOURCE | F

EYEBALL POINTS
V.10-11
(259-260) མྱིག་འབྲས་ཀྱི་གསང་།

LOCATION | One point on each side. Apply the appropriate form of moxa on the points located two fingers towards the forehead from the right and left Nest of Virus and Bacteria Point.

INDICATIONS |
* Burning sensation in the eyeballs
* Dryness and irritation of the eyes[139]
* Conjunctivitis[140]
* Hallucinations caused by contagious diseases

* Insanity

SOURCE | F

ANTERIOR FONTANEL POINT
V.12
(261) མཆོགས་མའི་གསང་།

LOCATION | One point. Apply the appropriate form of moxa on the point located two thumbs above the middle of the hairline.

INDICATIONS
* Migraine
* Dizziness
* Impaired vision
* Extreme forgetfulness
* Facial paresis affecting the mouth or nose (Wind-related)
* Swelling of the face
* Epilepsy

SOURCES | A, B, D, E, F, G

NOSE POINT
V.13
(262) སྣ་གསང་།

LOCATION | One point. Apply the appropriate form of moxa on the point located one thumb above the Anterior Fontanel Point.

INDICATIONS
* Nasal congestion
* Excessive nasal mucus that is difficult to expel

SOURCES | B, E

FOREHEAD POINT
V.14
(263) དཔྲལ་གསང་།

LOCATION | One point. Apply the appropriate form of moxa on the point located at the middle of the hairline on the forehead.

INDICATIONS
* Nasal congestion
* Excessive nasal mucus that is difficult to expel

SOURCES | B, C, D, E, F, G

Upper Eyebrow Points
V.15-16
(264-265) ཨྱེན་སྐྲང་གསང་།

LOCATION	One point on each side. Apply the appropriate form of moxa on the points located two fingers to the right and left of the Forehead Point.
INDICATIONS	• Eye illnesses in general • Eye illnesses related to a disturbance of Wind, Bile, or Phlegm humors • Eye problems such as irritation, tearing, redness, or burning (related to a combination of Blood and Wind)
SOURCE	F

Lateral Forehead Points
V.17-18
(266-267) དཔྲལ་བའི་ཟུར་གསང་།

LOCATION	One point on each side. Apply the appropriate form of moxa on the points located on the prominent bulge two thumbs to the right and left of the Forehead Point.
INDICATIONS	• Nosebleed (treat point on afflicted side)
SOURCE	E

Eye Points
V.19-20
(268-269) མིག་གསང་།

LOCATION	One point on each side. Apply the appropriate form of moxa on the points located one thumb below the hairline, directly over the eyeballs.
INDICATIONS	• Eye irritation[141] • Impaired vision • Migraine • Burning pain in the eyes
SOURCES	B, C, E

POINTS ABOVE THE EYEBROWS
V.21-22
(270-271)
སྨིན་གོང་གསང་།

LOCATION | One point on each side. Apply the appropriate form of moxa on the points located in the shallow area one thumb above the center of the eyebrows, directly over the pupil.

INDICATIONS |
* Facial swelling and burning sensation on the face (Wind-related)
* Dizziness
* Weak eyesight
* Severely impaired vision[142]

SOURCES | D, E

SHALLOW DIP POINT
V.23
(272)
ཞོང་མོའི་གསང་།

LOCATION | One point. Apply the appropriate form of moxa on the point located one thumb above the Point Between the Eyebrows.

INDICATIONS |
* Facial swelling (Wind-related), accompanied by an itching sensation as if insects were crawling on the skin
* Dizziness
* Weak eyesight
* Extreme forgetfulness
* Facial swelling
* Continuous nosebleed
* Impairment of the mental functions

SOURCES | B, C, D, E

POINT BETWEEN THE EYEBROWS
V.24
(273)
སྨིན་མཚམས་གསང་།

LOCATION | One point. Apply the appropriate form of moxa on the point located between the two eyebrows.

INDICATIONS |
* Eye illnesses
* Yellow complexion
* Yellow eyes
* Combined Blood and Wind disorders

- Brown Phlegm[143]
- Impaired vision
- Continuous nosebleed (resulting from exposure to heat or sun or insufficient sleep)
- Nasal congestion related to pulmonary diseases
- Combined Phlegm and Bile disorders
- Burning pain

SOURCES | B, C, D, E, F, G

EDGE OF THE EYEBROW POINTS
V.25-26 ཨྱེན་མཚག་གསང་།
(274-275)

LOCATION | One point on each side. Apply the appropriate form of moxa on the point located at the outer edge of each eyebrow where there is almost no hair.

INDICATIONS | • Ringing or roaring in the ears[144]
• Lacrimation

SOURCE | F

POSTERIOR EAR TIP POINTS
V.27-28 ཪྣ་ལྟག་གསང་།
(276-277)

LOCATION | One point on each side. Apply the appropriate form of moxa on the point on the head located at the level of the tip of each ear.

INDICATIONS | • Stiffness at the nape of the neck
• Stiffness on the sides of the neck

SOURCES | B, C, D, E

HELIX POINTS
V.29-30 ཪྣ་ཚག་གསང་།
(278-279)

LOCATION | One point on each side. Apply the appropriate form of moxa on the point located inside the helix at the tip of each ear.

INDICATIONS | • Loss of speech
• Dazed feeling

SOURCES | B, C, E

LATERAL EYE POINTS
V.31-32
(280-281)   ཨིག་ཟུར་གསང་།

LOCATION	One point on each side. Apply the appropriate form of moxa on the point located one thumb horizontally out from the corner of each eye.
INDICATIONS	• Eye irritation • Extreme forgetfulness • Impairment of the mental functions
SOURCES	B, C, E, G

HAIRLINE AT THE EAR POINTS
V.33-36
(282-285)   རྣ་བའི་སྐྲ་མཚམས་གསང་།

LOCATION	Two points on each side. Apply the appropriate form of moxa on the points located at the edge of the hairline near the temple close to the ears, on the front and behind.
INDICATIONS	• Earache • Pain in the nape of the neck • Migraine • Fainting
SOURCES	B, C, E

NASAL BRIDGE POINT
V.37
(286)   སྣ་འགྱིང་གསང་།

LOCATION	One point. Apply the appropriate form of moxa on the midline of the nasal bridge in the depression at the root of the nose.
INDICATIONS	• Surging pain in the facial bones • Toothache related to Wind[145] or caries[146] • Continuous nosebleed • Rhinitis • Nose tumors • Illnesses of the nose
SOURCES	D, F

FRONT OF THE EAR POINTS
V.38-39
(287-288) ཪ་རྡུང་གསང༌།

LOCATION	One point on each side. Apply the appropriate form of moxa on the points located in front of each ear.[147]
INDICATIONS	• Toothache (treat point on afflicted side) • Ringing in the ears
SOURCES	A, B, C, D, E, G

EYE PROXIMITY POINTS
V.40-43
(289-292) མིག་གི་ཉེ་གསང༌།

LOCATION	Two points on each side. Apply the appropriate form of moxa on the point located one thumb directly below the pupil of each eye and the point located one thumb below the outer corner of each eye.
INDICATIONS	• Blindness caused by early-stage edema associated with Phlegm[148]
SOURCES	E, G

TRAGUS POINTS
V.44-45
(293-294) ཪ་ཕུག་མདུན་གསང༌།

LOCATION	Two points on each side. Apply the appropriate form of moxa on the point located at the center of the shallow area above each tragus.
INDICATIONS	• Ringing in the ears • Toothache • Facial paresis (Wind-related) • Stiffness • Loss of hearing
SOURCES	A, B, C, D, E, G

FRONT EAR PROMINENCE POINTS
V.46-47
(295-296) ཪ་འབུར་གསང༌།

LOCATION	One point on each side. Apply the appropriate form of moxa on

the bony prominence located one finger in front of each ear at the level of the ear cavity.

INDICATIONS
- Inability to open the mouth due to glandular inflammation
- Inability to turn the head and neck to the right or left due to Wind or lymphatic disorders
- Eye irritation

SOURCES   B, C, D, E

BACK EAR PROMINENCE POINTS
V.48-49
(297-298)   ནེ་རྒྱབ་འབུར་གསང་།

LOCATION   One point on each side. Apply the appropriate form of moxa on the point located in the space or depression in the flesh behind the bony prominence in back of each helix.

INDICATIONS
- Inability to turn the head and neck to the right or left due to Wind or lymphatic disorders
- Eye irritation
- Ringing or roaring in the ears
- Passing of intestinal gas
- Ear illnesses
- Minor cerebral illnesses

SOURCE   F

EAR ARTERY POINTS
V.50-51
(299-300)   ནེ་འགྲུལ་གསང་།

LOCATION   One point on each side. Apply the appropriate form of moxa on the point located on the artery of each ear behind the anthelix.

INDICATIONS
- Headache
- Unclear state of mind
- Drowsiness and dazed feeling

SOURCES   B, C, E

EAR BONE POINTS

V.52-53
(301-302)

རྣ་རུས་གསང་།

LOCATION: One point on each side. Apply the appropriate form of moxa on the point located on the bony prominence one finger below the Back Ear Prominence Point on each side, away from the glands.

INDICATIONS:
- Speech difficulties
- Dropping of the lower jaw

SOURCE: F

GATE OF THE EAR POINTS

V.54-57
(303-306)

རྣ་སྒོའི་གསང་།

LOCATION: Two points on each side. Apply the appropriate form of moxa on the points in front of and behind each ear cavity.

INDICATIONS:
- Ringing in the ears
- Facial paresis (Wind-related)
- Drooling
- Stiffness
- Loss of hearing
- Problems with the jaws or teeth

SOURCES: B, C

POSTERIOR EAR CAVITY POINTS

V.58-59
(307-308)

རྣ་སུག་རྒྱབ་གསང་།

LOCATION: One point on each side. Apply the appropriate form of moxa on the point located in the depression in the flesh at the center of the bony prominence behind each ear.

INDICATIONS:
- Inability to turn the head and neck to the right or left due to Wind or lymphatic disorders
- Eye irritation
- Ringing or roaring in the ears
- Ear problems (Wind-related)
- Ear illnesses
- Minor cerebral illnesses

SOURCES | B, F

TIP OF THE NOSE POINT
V.60
(309) སྣ་རྩེའི་གསང༌།

LOCATION	One point. Apply the appropriate form of moxa on the indentation at the tip of the nose.
INDICATIONS	• Continuous nosebleed • Redness of the eyes caused by a hot condition • Injuries or swelling of the lips and nose • Swelling and pain in the penis
SOURCE	D

SMILE LINE POINTS
V.61-62
(310-311) ཁ་འགྱིང་གསང༌།

LOCATION	One point on each side. Apply the appropriate form of moxa on the point located two fingers away from the nose wings or the edge of the nose, perpendicular to the side of the mouth.
INDICATIONS	• Facial paresis affecting the mouth or nose • Skin diseases
SOURCE	F

CHEEK POINTS
V.63-64
(312-313) མཁུར་ཚོས་གསང༌།

LOCATION	One point on each side. Apply the appropriate form of moxa on the point located at the center of each cheek.
INDICATIONS	• Facial paresis (Wind-related) • Stiffness • Loss of hearing
SOURCE	D

JAW POINTS
V.65-66
(314-315)   ཟ་འགྲམ་གསང་།

LOCATION	One point on each side. Apply the appropriate form of moxa on the point located on the jaw at the level of each earlobe.
INDICATIONS	• Inability to open the mouth • Facial paresis affecting the mouth or eyes • Facial paresis and swelling (Wind-related) • Toothache in the upper teeth related to Wind or caries • Loss of speech • Loss of hearing
SOURCES	B, C, D, E, G

UPPER LIP POINT
V.67
(316)   མཆུ་གོང་གསང་།

LOCATION	One point. Apply the appropriate form of moxa on the point located in the philtrum above the upper lip.
INDICATIONS	• Loss of speech or speech impairments related to contagious diseases associated with Wind disorders • Impairment of the mental functions • Delirious speech
SOURCE	E

ROOT OF THE TEETH POINTS
V.68-69
(317-318)   སོ་རྩའི་གསང་།

LOCATION	One point on each side. Apply the appropriate form of moxa on the point located one thumb above each side of the mouth.
INDICATIONS	• Facial paresis affecting the mouth • Facial paresis affecting the eyes • Surging pain in the jaws (Wind-related) • Toothache related to caries and other dental problems
SOURCES	B, C, D, E, F, G

TONGUE POINTS

V.70-71 (319-320) ལྕེ་གསང་།

LOCATION One point on each side. Apply the appropriate form of moxa on the point located at the side of the mouth or one thumb below the Root of the Teeth Point.

INDICATIONS

- Bitter taste in the mouth
- Swelling at the root of the tongue
- Angina
- Bone tumors
- Tongue tumors
- Stuttering
- Illnesses of the tongue

SOURCES B, C, E, F, G

LOWER LIP POINT

V.72 (321) མཆུ་འོག་གསང་།

LOCATION One point. Apply the appropriate form of moxa on the depressed area below the lower lip.

INDICATIONS

- Loss of speech
- Speech difficulties resulting from severe mouth ulcers
- Impairment of the mental functions
- Drowsiness and fogginess
- Delirious speech
- Conditions related to contamination or provocations
- Loss of speech as a result of contagious diseases associated with Wind disorders
- Throat illnesses

SOURCES A, B, C, D, E, F, G

CHIN POINT

V.73 (322) ཀོས་གསང་།

LOCATION One point. Apply the appropriate form of moxa on the dimple of the chin.

INDICATIONS	• Stuttering
	• Speech impairments
	• Swelling of the tongue
SOURCE	E

OCCIPITAL LIGAMENT POINT
V.74
(323)   ལྷག་འཆུའི་གསང༌།

LOCATION	One point. Apply the appropriate form of moxa on the point located at the center of the depression between the occipital ligaments.
INDICATIONS	• Insanity and impairment of the mental functions (Wind-related)
	• Dizziness
	• Stiffness at the back of the head
	• Numbness or tingling
	• Continuous nosebleed
SOURCES	B, C, D, E

OCCIPITAL PROTUBERANCE POINT
V.75
(324)   ལྷག་འབུར་གསང༌།

LOCATION	One point. Apply the appropriate form of moxa on the point located on the bulging protuberance of the occipital bone.
INDICATIONS	• Dizziness and pain in the head (Wind-related)
	• Drowsiness caused by contagious diseases
	• Impairment of the brain functions or brain injury
SOURCE:	D

UPPER OCCIPITAL POINT
V.76
(325)   ལྷག་གོང་གསང༌།

LOCATION	One point. Apply the appropriate form of moxa on the point located one thumb above the occipital protuberance.
INDICATIONS	• Nasal congestion
	• Unclear vision

- Impaired vision
- Cerebrospinal fluid disorders (related to a combination of Blood, Bile, and lymph)
- Drowsiness and headaches caused by fever, Wind-related provocations, combined Blood and Bile disorders, or a major disturbance of one's physical condition
- Vertigo and sensation that the head is spinning during movement
- Vertigo and sensation of falling over when leaning
- Illnesses related to combined Phlegm and Wind disorders or an abnormal blood condition

SOURCES | B, C, E, F

BRAIN POINTS
V.77-78
(326-327) གྲད་གསང་།

LOCATION | One point. Apply the appropriate form of moxa on the points located one thumb directly to the right and left of the Upper Occipital Point.

INDICATIONS |
- Eye illnesses
- Nosebleeds
- Thickening of the cerebral membrane[149]

SOURCES | B, C, D, E

GATE OF UNION POINT
V.79
(328) སྡུད་སྒོའི་གསང་།

LOCATION | One point. Apply the appropriate form of moxa on the "Gate of Union," or posterior occipital fontanel, at the same level as the tip of the ear.

INDICATIONS |
- Cardiac complaints caused by virulent contagious fever
- Numbness or tingling
- Yellow eyes
- Provocations related to the planets[150]
- Wind disorders caused by contamination
- Dizziness related to combined Phlegm and Bile disorders
- Frequent yawning

* Epilepsy

SOURCES | A, B, C, D, E, F, G

OCCIPITAL WHORL POINTS
V.80-81
(329-330) ལྕུག་འཁྱིལ་གཉིས།

LOCATION | One point on each side. Apply the appropriate form of moxa on the points located on the hairline whorl on each side of the occipital region, where firm pressure triggers a darting pain in the eyes.

INDICATIONS |
* Stiffness of the neck
* Numbness in the nape of the neck
* Tension in the nape of the neck
* Surging pain in the nape of the neck
* Conditions related to contamination or provocations
* Fainting
* Insanity and seizures
* Provocations from above[151]
* Sudden pain of unidentified origin

SOURCES | A, E, G

These constitute the eighty-one most important and most effective moxa points of the head.

VI. POINTS ON THE ARMS

There are eighty-four major moxa points on the arms that are particularly effective. These points are listed and described below.

POINTS BETWEEN THE SHOULDER AND NECK

VI.1-2
(331-332) ཕྲག་ཐལ་གསང་།

LOCATION	One point on each side. Apply the appropriate form of moxa on the point located on the top of each shoulder, about midway between the shoulder and neck joint.
INDICATIONS	• Angina • Illnesses of the larynx • Swelling of the larynx • Pulmonary diseases • Inability to raise the arms • Upper back pain
SOURCES	B, C, E, G

UPPER SHOULDER POINTS

VI.3-4
(333-334) དཔུང་ཕྲག་གསང་།

LOCATION	One point on each side. Apply the appropriate form of moxa on the point located where the breath falls on the top of the shoulder.[152]
INDICATIONS	• Profuse nosebleed
SOURCES	A, B, C, E, G

SHOULDER DEPRESSION POINTS

VI.5-6
(335-336) དཔུང་ག་ཤོང་གསང་།

LOCATION	One point on each side. Apply the appropriate form of moxa on the point located in the middle of the depression on each upper shoulder.[153]
INDICATIONS	• Problems with the joints such as accumulation of lymph • Barking cough • Blood obstructions such as thrombosis[154]

- Nerve disorders
- Swellings (Wind-related)

SOURCES | B, C, D, E, F

UPPER ARM CURVE POINTS
VI.7-8
(337-338) དཔུང་འཛུམ་གསང༌།

LOCATION | One point on each side. Apply the appropriate form of moxa on the point located half a finger in the direction of the top of each shoulder from Points II.31 and II.32 on the lateral back,[155] mentioned in Dilmar's *White Crystal*.

INDICATIONS |
- Lameness in the arms
- Eye impairments[156]
- Nosebleed

SOURCES | E, G

SHOULDER BLADE POINTS
VI.9-10
(339-340) སྐྱོག་རའི་གསང༌།

LOCATION | One point on each side. Apply the appropriate form of moxa on the point located at the apex of the projecting oblong bone on each shoulder blade.

INDICATIONS |
- Partial blindness

SOURCE | E

BACK SHOULDER JOINT POINTS
VI.11-12
(341-342) དཔུང་ཚིགས་ཕྱི་ལྟེའི་གསང༌།

LOCATION | One point on each side. Apply the appropriate form of moxa on the point located at the center of the articulation of each shoulder joint on the back.

INDICATIONS |
- Excessive movement of the joints
- Sensation of laxity of the joints
- Frozen shoulder
- Painful dry cough
- Illnesses caused by an accumulation of lymph

SOURCES | B, C, D

FRONT SHOULDER JOINT POINTS
VI.13-14
(343-344)
དཔུང་ཚིགས་ནང་ལྩོའི་གསང་།

LOCATION | One point on each side. Apply the appropriate form of moxa on the point located at the center of the articulation of each shoulder joint at the front.

INDICATIONS |
* Excessive movement of the joints
* Sensation of laxity of the joints
* Frozen shoulder
* Painful dry cough
* Illnesses caused by an accumulation of lymph

SOURCES | B, C, D

CREASE OF THE ARMPIT POINTS
VI.15-16
(345-346)
མཆན་གཉེར་གསང་།

LOCATION | One point on each side. Apply the appropriate form of moxa on the point located at the top of the long crease behind each armpit.

INDICATIONS |
* Tightness and heaviness in the upper back
* Lameness in the arms

SOURCES | B, C, E

BACK OF THE UPPER ARM POINTS
VI.17-22
(347-352)
དཔུང་རྒྱབ་གསང་།

LOCATION | Three points on each side. Apply the appropriate form of moxa on the two groups of three points on the back of each arm: the first set of points is located two fingers below the depression in the flesh where the tendons of the shoulder converge with the tendons of the upper arm; the second set two fingers below that; and the third two fingers below that.

INDICATION |
* Facial paresis (Wind-related)
* Stiffness
* Loss of hearing
* Nerve problems (Wind-related)

- Abnormal presence of lymph in the vascular system[155]
- Mottled skin
- Lymph affecting tissue between the flesh and nerves

SOURCES | D, F

BENT BOW POINTS
VI.23-24
(353-354) ᡍᠵᡠᢖᡠᢛᢐᢛᢐ᠎᠎᠎᠎᠎᠎᠎᠎᠎

LOCATION | One point on each side. Apply the appropriate form of moxa on the point located in the indentation above the bent bow or rounded curvature above the elbow on the back of each arm.[158]

INDICATIONS | All types of bone diseases

SOURCE | C

UPPER ARM ARTERY POINTS
VI.25-26
(355-356) ᡏᢖᢛᡏᡎᡏᢖᢛᡏ

LOCATION | One point on each side. Apply the appropriate form of moxa on the point located on the bulge toward the back of each elbow where the pulse of the artery connecting the shoulder and the forearm can be felt.

INDICATIONS |
- Pain in the arms
- Arm problems caused by pulmonary lymph
- Excessive movement of the elbow joint
- Edema swelling (Wind-related)[159]
- Pain in the sides of the torso in females
- Pulmonary diseases in males

SOURCES | B, C, D

FOLD OF THE ELBOW POINTS
VI.27-28
(357-358) ᡍᢖᡏᢖᢛᡏ

LOCATION | One point on each side. Apply the appropriate form of moxa on the point located in the fold of each elbow.

INDICATIONS | All illnesses caused by lymphatic disorders

SOURCES | B, C, E

ELBOW POINTS
VI.29-30
(359-360) གྲུ་འབུར་གསང་།

LOCATION | One point on each side. Apply the appropriate form of moxa on the bony prominence of each elbow.

INDICATIONS | ° Joint problems
° Bone problems

SOURCES | B, E

BOW JOINT POINTS
VI.31-34
(361-364) གཞུ་ཚིགས་གསང་།

LOCATION | Two points on each side. Apply the appropriate form of moxa on the two points located directly to the right and left of each elbow joint.

INDICATIONS | ° Neuralgia
° Lameness
° Contraction of the tendons

SOURCE | E

LOWER ELBOW POINTS
VI.35-36
(365-366) གྲུ་དར་འཆུ་གསང་།

LOCATION | One point on each side. Apply the appropriate form of moxa on the point located one finger below the elbow joint on the back of each forearm.

INDICATIONS | ° Facial paresis (Wind-related)
° Stiffness
° Loss of hearing
° Surging pain and numbness or tingling in the legs
° Internal or external lymphatic disorders causing pain in the flesh and skin[160]
° Wind disorders caused by contamination
° Muscular cramps and spasms related to gout or arthritis

SOURCES | D, F

WRIST TENDON POINTS
VI.37-38
(367-368)   མ་ཁྲིག་འཆུའི་གསང་།

LOCATION | One point on each side. Apply the appropriate form of moxa on the point located between the tendons on each inner forearm, four fingers above the wrist.

INDICATIONS |
- Contagious diseases accompanied by sobbing
- Hallucinations and logorrhea
- Vomiting
- Stiffness at the back of the head
- Weak eyesight
- Bone problems
- Continuous nosebleed

SOURCES | A, B, C, E, G

FOREARM TENDON POINTS
VI.39-48
(369-378)   གླུ་ངར་འཆུ་རྒྱུད་གསང་།

LOCATION | Five points on each side. Apply the appropriate form of moxa on the five points located on the depression in the flesh between the tendons on each outer forearm, starting at the point five fingers above the wrist. The second point is two fingers from the first, and the others are one finger apart from each other.

INDICATIONS |
- Facial paresis (Wind-related)
- Stiffness
- Loss of hearing
- Surging pain and numbness or tingling in the legs
- Internal or external lymphatic disorders causing pain in the flesh and skin[161]
- Wind disorders caused by contamination
- Muscular cramps and spasms related to gout or arthritis

SOURCE | F

ULNAR WRIST POINTS
VI.49-50
(379-380)
མ་ཁྲིག་འབུར་གསང་།

LOCATION	One point on each side. Apply the appropriate form of moxa on the point located on the ulna bone on each wrist.
INDICATIONS	• Warts and other skin problems[162]
SOURCES	B, C, E, G

RADIAL WRIST POINTS
VI.51-52
(381-382)
མ་ཐེབ་མ་ཁྲིག་ལོང་བུའི་གསང་།

LOCATION	One point on each side. Apply the appropriate form of moxa on the point located on the prominence on the thumb side of each wrist.
INDICATIONS	• Cerebral illnesses • Eye illnesses
SOURCES	B, E

WRIST CREASE POINTS
VI.53-58
(383-388)
མ་ཁྲིག་གཉིར་གསང་།

LOCATION	Three points on each side. Apply the appropriate form of moxa on the three points located one finger apart from each other along the long crease on each inner wrist.
INDICATIONS	• Loss of speech as a result of contagious diseases • Dryness of the lower lip • Stiffness of the tendons and ligaments
SOURCES	B, C

LATERAL WRIST POINTS
VI.59-60
(389-390)
མ་ཁྲིག་ཟུར་གསང་།

LOCATION	One point on each side. Apply the appropriate form of moxa on the point located on the vein on the little finger side of the wrist on the back of each hand.

INDICATIONS	• Stiffness of the tendons and ligaments • Contraction of the tendons and ligaments
SOURCES	B, E

CROOK OF THE WRIST POINTS
VI.61-62
(391-392)
 མ་ཐེབ་མ་ཁྲིག་གི་འོང་གསང་།

LOCATION	One point on each side. Apply the appropriate form of moxa on the point located in the crook between each wrist and thumb.
INDICATIONS	• Cerebral illnesses • Lacrimation
SOURCES	B, C, E

FOREARM CONCAVITY POINT
VI.63-64
(393-394)
ལག་དར་སྲུབ་གསང་།

LOCATION	One point on each side. Apply the appropriate form of moxa on the point located in the concavity in the flesh six fingers from the web between each thumb and index finger.
INDICATIONS	• Facial paresis (Wind-related) • Stiffness • Loss of hearing • Internal or external lymphatic disorders causing pain in the flesh and skin[163] • Wind disorders caused by contamination • Muscular cramps and spasms related to gout or arthritis
SOURCE	E

THUMB/INDEX POINTS
VI.65-66
(395-396)
མ་ཐེབ་མཛུབ་གསང་།

LOCATION	One point on each side. Apply the appropriate form of moxa on the point located one thumb from the web between the thumb and the index fingers on each hand.
INDICATIONS	• Contagious fever • Eye illnesses related to fevers

SOURCES | B, C, D, E, G

LITTLE/RING FINGER POINTS
VI.67-68
(397-398)
མཐེའུ་སྲིན་གསང་།

LOCATION | One point on each side. Apply the appropriate form of moxa on the point located one thumb and one finger from the web between the little and ring finger on each hand.

INDICATIONS | • Eye cysts or sties
• Eye irritation

SOURCES | B, C, E, G

FINGER JUNCTION POINTS
VI.69-74
(399-404)
མཐེའུ་མཚོབ་མདོ་གསང་།

LOCATION | Three points on each side. Apply the appropriate form of moxa on the three points located between the knuckles of the four main fingers on each hand.

INDICATIONS | • Swelling and pain in the arms caused by lung edema[164]
• Continuous cough and respiratory problems
• Lymph flowing in between the joints of the limbs
• Teeth problems caused by Wind disorders

SOURCE | D

RING FINGER POINTS
VI.75-80
(405-410)
སྲིན་ཚིགས་གསང་།

LOCATION | One, two, or three points on each side. Depending on the seriousness of the problem, apply the appropriate form of moxa on one, two, or three of the joints of the ring finger on the back of each hand. The principal point is on the middle joint.

INDICATIONS | • Swelling of the lips
• Illnesses caused by an accumulation of Phlegm

SOURCES | A, E, G

TIP OF THE INDEX FINGER POINT
VI.81-82
(411-412) མཛུབ་སྟེའི་གསང་།

LOCATION	One point on each side. Apply the appropriate form of moxa on the point located on the tip of each index finger.
INDICATIONS	• Yellow eyes • Increase of Bile • Sudden surging bone pain • Toothache related to Wind or caries • Gum or teeth problems resulting from parasites or bacteria
SOURCE	D

TIP OF THE RING FINGER POINTS
VI.83-84
(413-414) སྲིན་ལག་རྩེ་གསང་།

LOCATION	One point on each side. Apply the appropriate form of moxa on the tip of each ring finger.
INDICATIONS	• Toothache (treat point on afflicted side)
SOURCES	A, E, G

These constitute the eighty-four most important and most effective moxa points on the arms.

VII. POINTS ON THE LEGS

There are eighty-six moxa points on the legs that are particularly effective. These are listed and described below.

ROOT OF THE HIP POINTS
VII.1-2
(415-416) དཔྱི་ཙྩེའི་གསང་།

LOCATION	One point on each side. Apply the appropriate form of moxa on the point located three thumbs above the prominence on the upper extremity of the femur on each side.
INDICATIONS	• Swelling of the calf • Numbness or tingling in the legs • Illnesses affecting the legs in general
SOURCES	B, C, E, G

HIP PROTUBERANCE POINTS
VII.3-4
(417-418) དཔྱི་འབུར་གསང་།

LOCATION	One point on each side. Apply the appropriate form of moxa on the point located on the prominence on the upper extremity of the femur on each side.
INDICATIONS	• Wind or lymphatic disorders affecting the inner parts of the body • Cold sensation in the lower torso • Localized pain and inability to lift the lower body as a result of major and minor Wind disorders affecting the joints • Formation of lymph in the kidneys • Impotence resulting from excessive sexual intercourse • Edema swelling[165]
SOURCES	B, D, F

LATERAL HIP POINTS
VII.5-6
(419-420) དཔྱི་ཟུར་གསང་།

LOCATION	One point on each side. Apply the appropriate form of moxa on the point located four fingers and one thumb behind each hip

joint.[166] This point is evident when one sits in the cross-legged posture with the body straight and hands in the meditation gesture.

INDICATIONS
* Sensation of heat and pain in the feet causing inability to walk[167]
* Surging pain in the lumbar joints

SOURCES | B, C, E

HOLLOW OF THE HIP POINTS
VII.7-8 དཔྱི་ག་ཤོང་གསང་།
(421-422)

LOCATION | One point on each side. Apply the appropriate form of moxa on the point located in the hollow area on each thigh below the prominence at the upper extremity of the femur.

INDICATIONS
* Lymph descending into the inner parts of the body
* Edema caused by tumors of a cold nature[168]
* Dry stools

SOURCES | B, C, E

SIDE OF THE THIGH POINTS
VII.9-10 བརླ་སྒུལ་གསང་།
(423-424)

LOCATION | One point on each side. Apply the appropriate form of moxa on the point on each thigh where the middle finger reaches when one stands upright with the arms straight down and aligned next to the side of the thigh.

INDICATIONS
* Lumbar pain
* Lameness in the legs
* Surging pain in the legs
* Pain in the thighs
* Instability in the lower body
* Leg problems causing difficulty in walking and sitting

SOURCES | A, B, C, D, E, G

THIGH MUSCLE DEPRESSION POINTS
VII.11-12
(425-426)
གཉག་གཞོང་གོང་གསང་།

LOCATION	One point on each side. Apply the appropriate form of moxa on the point located on the front of each thigh at the level of the Side of the Thigh Point.
INDICATIONS	• Pain in the legs • Surging pain in the bones of the legs • Inability to lift the lower body • Problems related to the lower body in general
SOURCES	B, C, E

POINTS ABOVE THE KNEECAP
VII.13-14
(427-428)
ཕྱུང་ཕྱུག་གསང་།

LOCATION	One point on each side. Apply the appropriate form of moxa on the point located four fingers up from the upper edge of each kneecap with the leg fully extended.
INDICATIONS	• Emaciated legs • Problems in the lumbar region • Gynecological disorders • Risk of miscarriage • Infertility
SOURCES	B, C, E

POINTS ABOVE THE KNEE
VII.15-18
(429-432)
པུས་གོང་གསང་།

LOCATION	Two points on each side. Apply the appropriate form of moxa on the two points located four fingers above the right and left side of each knee.
INDICATIONS	• Wind disorders affecting the joints • Surging pain in the upper knees caused by lymph • Dislocation of the knee joints • Blockage of the patella • Leg problems causing difficulties when walking, sitting, and

stretching or bending the legs

SOURCES | D, F

SIDE OF THE KNEECAP POINTS
VII.19-20
(433-434)   སྐྱི་མཆུན་གསང་།

LOCATION | One point on each side. Apply the appropriate form of moxa on the point located on the inner front side of each kneecap, one thumb plus one finger from the long crease that is evident when the knee is bent.

INDICATIONS | ° Pain in the knee joints causing inability to walk
° Numbness or tingling and pain in the hip joints
° Swelling of the penis
° Fleshy growths[169]

SOURCES | B, C, D, E

BACK OF KNEE POINTS
VII.21-22
(435-436)   ཕྱིན་ཁུག་གསང་།

LOCATION | One point on each side. Apply the appropriate form of moxa on the point located on the back of each knee on the bulge formed by the tendons and ligaments that can be felt with the hand when the legs are extended.

INDICATIONS | ° Kidney disorders
° Lymph affecting the legs
° Pain in the spleen
° Accumulation of lymph in the back of the legs

SOURCE | D

POINTS BELOW THE KNEECAP
VII.23-24
(437-438)   སྐྱི་འོག་གསང་།

LOCATION | One point on each side. Apply the appropriate form of moxa on the point called the Eye of the Crow, located in the depression directly below each kneecap.[170]

INDICATIONS | ° Cold sensation in the stomach

- Poor digestion
- Weak eyesight
- Impaired vision
- Surging pain in the calf

SOURCES | B, C, E

LATERAL POINTS BELOW THE KNEECAP
VII.25-28
(439-442)   ལྕུང་ཁའི་འོག་གསང་།

LOCATION | Two points on each side. Apply the appropriate form of moxa on the points located on the right and left sides of the knee joint one thumb below the center of each kneecap.

INDICATIONS |
- Inability to digest food
- Numbness or tingling in the legs at the knees and below
- Pain in the bones around the eyes
- Pain in the calf
- Surging pain from swellings

SOURCES | B, C, E

KNEE CREASE POINTS
VII.29-30
(443-444)   སྙིད་ག་ཉེར་འོག་གསང་།

LOCATION | One point on each side. Apply the appropriate form of moxa on the point located one thumb below the long crease at the back of each knee.

INDICATIONS |
- Contraction of the tendons
- Inability to stretch the legs
- Hemorrhoids

SOURCES | B, C, D, E

TENDON GAP POINTS
VII.31-32
(445-446)   འཆུ་དབྲག་གསང་།

LOCATION | One point on each side. Apply the appropriate form of moxa on the point also known as the Major Heart Channel Point, located in the gap between the tendons at the upper shin.

INDICATIONS
- Intestinal problems
- Yellow complexion
- Yellow eyes
- Swelling of the abdomen and liver
- Swelling of the penis
- Retraction of the testicles

SOURCES | B, C, E

KNEECAP TENDON POINTS
VII.33-34
(447-448) ལྔད་འཁྱུའི་གསང་ད།

LOCATION | One point on each side. Apply the appropriate form of moxa on the point located in the gap between the tendons and ligaments that is evident when the leg is bent.

INDICATIONS
- Lymph affecting the lower body
- Heaviness of the legs
- Swelling of the larynx
- Pain in the kidneys and lumbar region and below
- Priapism accompanied by walking difficulties

SOURCES | B, C, D

SHANK POINTS
VII.35-36
(449-450) རྗེ་དར་གསང་ད།

LOCATION | One point on each side. Apply the appropriate form of moxa on the point located on each shank, six fingers below the prominence at the top of the shinbone (referred to as the blind eye).

INDICATIONS
- Bleeding between menstrual periods

SOURCES | B, C, E

MUSCLE DEPRESSION POINTS
VII.37-38
(451-452) གནག་ག་གལོང་གསང་ད།

LOCATION | One point on each side. Apply the appropriate form of moxa on the point located in the depression at the end of the muscle on the lateral side of each shinbone. My sublime master explained this point to me in person.

INDICATIONS
- Pain in the legs
- Surging pain in the bones of the legs
- Inability to lift the lower body
- All other problems with the lower body

SOURCES B, C, E

Shank Tendon Points

VII.39-40
(453-454)
གདོང་འཁྱུའི་གསང་།

LOCATION One point on each side. Apply the appropriate form of moxa on the point located between the shin tendons on the inside of each leg (midway up the lower leg), straight up from the ankle bone.

INDICATIONS
- Impairment of the male sexual organ
- Impotence
- Loss and leakage of semen

SOURCES B, C, E

Cleft in the Calf Points

VII.41-46
(455-460)
ཉ་སྐྱབས་གསང་།

LOCATION Three points on each side. According to the medical text called *The Continuous Rainfall of Nectar,*[171] this group actually consists of six points on each leg, each two fingers from the other, starting on the calf four fingers below the center of the back of the knee. However, the first set of points is identical to the Knee Crease Points.[172] Among the remaining five sets of points on each leg, my sacred master said that the third, fourth, and fifth are particularly effective. Accordingly, apply the appropriate form of moxa on these six points.[173]

INDICATIONS
- Edema[174]
- Pain in the kidneys and lumbar region
- Pain in the lungs
- Trembling of the calves
- Dislocation of the leg joints
- Nerve disorders

- Vascular conditions
- Lymphatic disorders
- Gout
- Arthritis, rheumatism
- Vascular conditions (Wind-related)
- Dispersion or concentration of pure blood
- Problems in the joints caused by lymph or impure blood
- Accumulation of liquid in the joints

SOURCES | D, F

HEEL ARTERY POINTS
VII.47-48
(461-462)   ཏིང་འཆུའི་འགུལ་གསང་།

LOCATION | One point on each side. Apply the appropriate form of moxa on the point located on the pulsating artery at each heel.[175]

INDICATIONS |
- Frequent nausea
- Lack of appetite
- Diarrhea
- Bleeding between menstrual periods
- Swelling of the larynx

SOURCES | B, C, E

MEDIAL TENDON POINTS
VII.49-50
(463-464)   ནང་འཆུའི་གསང་།

LOCATION | One point on each side. Apply the appropriate form of moxa on the point located one thumb above the medial malleolus of each ankle.

INDICATIONS | • Continuous menstruation

SOURCE | E

SHANK DECLIVITY POINTS
VII.51-52
(465-466)   སྤྱར་མགོའི་གསང་།

LOCATION | One point on each side. Apply the appropriate form of moxa on the point located just below the round bone at the lower extremity of each shank.

INDICATIONS

- Surging pain in the bones of the legs
- Muscular spasms in the calves
- Problems above and below the knees

SOURCES B, C, E

JOINT OF THE FOOT POINTS
VII.53-54
467-468)

རྐང་མགུལ་གསང་།

LOCATION

One point on each side. Apply the appropriate form of moxa on the point located between the tendons and ligaments at the lower extremity of each shin, on the joint that moves the top of the foot.

INDICATIONS

- Aggravation and spreading of hot or cold conditions
- Acute spreading of cold conditions
- Lack of kidney heat due to cold or extreme cold
- Swelling of the testicles
- Loss of semen
- Bleeding between menstrual periods

SOURCE F

TOE INDENTATION POINTS
VII.55-56
(469-470)

མཛུབ་སྤུབས་གསང་།

LOCATION

One point on each side. Apply the appropriate form of moxa on the point located in the indentation in the flesh on the top of each foot, three fingers from the joint of the foot.

INDICATIONS

- Gout
- Arthritis, rheumatism
- Edema caused by lymphatic disorders[176]
- Severe edema[177]

SOURCE F

PENIS POINTS

VII.57-58 (471-472) རྨིག་གསང་།

LOCATION	One point on each side. Apply the appropriate form of moxa on the point located three thumbs above the space in between the big toe and the second toe on each foot.
INDICATIONS	• Sensation of heaviness • Swelling of the penis
SOURCES	B, C, E

MEDIAL MALLEOLUS POINTS

VII.59-60 (473-474) ནང་ལོང་གསང་།

LOCATION	One point on each side. Apply the appropriate form of moxa on the artery on the side of the medial malleolus on the inside of each foot.
INDICATIONS	• Disorders of the small and large intestines • Colic • Wind disorders affecting the joints
SOURCES	A, D, E, G

TOP OF THE FOOT POINTS

VII.61-62 (475-476) རྡོལ་གསང་།

LOCATION	One point on each side. Apply the appropriate form of moxa on the point located directly above the third toe on the central upper part of each foot.
INDICATIONS	• Inability to stand • Swelling of the legs • Facial swelling (Wind-related), accompanied by an itching sensation as if insects were crawling on the skin • Sensation as if the body were sinking and vertigo • Weak eyesight
SOURCES	B, C, D, E

BIG TOE LIGAMENT POINTS
VII.63-64
(477-478)   མཐེབ་རྒྱུས་ཀྱི་གསང་།

LOCATION	One point on each side. Apply the appropriate form of moxa on the point located on the tendons and ligaments four fingers above the tip of each big toe, measured while standing erect with the heels placed on the ground.
INDICATIONS	° Contagious fever concentrated in the head ° Pain when moving the neck to the right or left ° Ear problems (Wind-related)
SOURCE	D

BIG TOE INDENTATION POINTS
VII.65-66
(479-480)   མཐེབ་གཤོང་གསང་།

LOCATION	One point on each side. Apply the appropriate form of moxa on the point located in the indentation at the top of each big toe, evident when the toes are contracted.
INDICATIONS	° Cerebral illnesses ° Urine retention ° Swelling of the penis
SOURCES	B, C, E

BIG TOE JOINT POINTS
VII.67-68
(481-482)   མཐེབ་ཚིགས་གསང་།

LOCATION	One point on each side. Apply the appropriate form of moxa on the joint of each big toe.
INDICATIONS	° Gout
SOURCES	B, C, D, E, G

BIG AND SECOND TOE INDENTATION POINTS
VII.69-70
(483-484)   མཐེབ་མཛུབ་གཤོང་གསང་།

LOCATION	One point on each side. Apply the appropriate form of moxa on the point located one thumb above the space between the big toe

and second toe on each foot.

INDICATIONS
- Cerebral illnesses
- Numbness or tingling in the legs
- Lymphatic disorders
- Large belly
- Urine retention
- Lame and arthritic thighs and legs
- Sensation of heat and pain in the feet causing inability to walk
- Swelling of the penis

SOURCES   B, C, E

TOE TENDON POINTS
VII.71-76
(485-490)   མཛུབ་འཆུའི་གསང་།

LOCATION   Three points on each side. Apply the appropriate form of moxa on the points located in the gaps between the tendons and ligaments between the small, third, and second toes on each foot.

INDICATIONS
- Surging pain caused by fever
- Edema caused by lymphatic disorders[178]
- Heaviness and instability of the legs and surging pain during movement[179]
- Inability to bend the body backward and forward
- Joint problems
- Residual gout and arthritis

SOURCES   D, F

BIG TOE POINTS
VII.77-78
(491-492)   ཀྲང་མཐེབ་གསང་།

LOCATION   One point on each side. Apply the appropriate form of moxa on the point located where the hair grows on each big toe.[180]

INDICATIONS
- Insanity and seizures
- Loss of speech
- Stiffness at the back of the head
- Swelling of the penis

SOURCES   A, E, G

HEEL DEPRESSION POINTS
VII.79-80
(493-494)   ཏིང་ག་ཤོང་གསང་།

LOCATION	One point on each side. Apply the appropriate form of moxa on the point located in the depression above the heel bone at the back of each foot.
INDICATIONS	• Pain in the legs • Pain in the calf • Pain behind the knees
SOURCE	E

HEEL POINTS
VII.81-82
(495-496)   ཏིང་གསང་།

LOCATION	One point on each side. Apply the appropriate form of moxa on the point located between the rough and smooth skin at the back of each heel.
INDICATIONS	• Eye irritation • Seizures due to swellings • Locking of the jaw • Bubbles forming at the corner of the eyes • Insanity and seizures • Psychosis • Conditions related to provocations
SOURCES	A, B, C, E, G

DEPRESSION OF THE LATERAL MALLEOLUS POINTS
VII.83-84
(497-498)   ཕྱི་ལོང་ག་ཤོང་གསང་།

LOCATION	One point on each side. Apply the appropriate form of moxa on the point located in the depression below the bony prominence of the lateral malleolus on each ankle.
INDICATIONS	• Pain in the legs • Pain in the calf • Pain behind the knees
SOURCES	B, C, D

SOLE OF THE FOOT POINTS
VII.85-86
(499-500)   ཀང་མཐིལ་གསང་།

LOCATION	One point on each side. Apply the appropriate form of moxa on the point located in the middle of the sole of each foot, midway between the tip of the third toe and the heel.
INDICATIONS	• Lymphatic disorders • Leg problems • Eye problems[181]
SOURCES	C, E

These constitute the eighty-six most effective moxa points on the legs.

SUMMARY

The purpose of this concise manual on moxa is to promote good health and cure the various kinds of illnesses that affect the different parts of the bodies of adults, children, and the elderly, both male and female. The text covers the five hundred most effective points for moxa therapy and clearly explains the various indications and their healing benefits.

Concluding Verses

This precious treasure
Of five hundred crucial moxa points,
The quintessence of the supreme therapy
Of the practice of moxa,
Has been presented here
As an ornament of the healing art
Of Shang Shung and Tibet.

May the light of the newly risen sun
Of the practice of moxa
Gently illuminate the clear and limpid surface
Of the pure crystal mirror of my intentions,
Dispelling the frost
Of hot and cold illnesses of beings,
And may the lotus grove,
Wealth of happiness and well-being,
Blossom!

Invoked by the white aurora
Of the merit of this good deed,
May myriad suns of myriad virtues
Rise and forever shine in our world,
For all, without distinction,
Eradicating negative actions,
Passions, and obscurity!

AFTERWORD

I, Chögyal Namkhai Norbu, composed this text, originally entitled *The Clear Crystal Mirror*, to facilitate the practice of moxibustion in day-to-day life. It is a condensed compilation from a larger text called *Graced with Seven Excellencies*, an ongoing comparison undertaken during years of research of several important Tibetan medical texts on moxibustion: *The Last Tantra*; *The Moon King*, a translation from the Sanskrit; *Somaraja*, a translation from the Chinese; two medical books on moxibustion found among the ancient manuscripts of Tun-Huang; *The White Crystal Mirror: An Extensive Instruction Manual on Moxibustion*, written by Dilmar; *The Continuous Rainfall of Nectar That Preserves the Life of Beings*, an extraordinary medical treatise offering methods for curing illnesses of our era discovered as a hidden treasure by my root master, the incomparable knowledge holder Changchub Dorje; and *The Excellent Wish-Fulfilling Tree: An Indispensable Ornament of the Quintessence of Myriad Treatises on the Art of Healing*, written by the Shang Shung doctor Khyungchen Pungri Khyungtrul Jigme Namkhai Dorje Yungdrung Gyaltsan. Those wishing to learn in greater detail should refer to these books.

With the hope of developing the practice of Tibetan medicine, ignoring difficulties and accepting fatigue, I have persevered for many years conducting research on moxibustion therapy. What is presented here is a drop, a mere fraction, of the moxibustion therapies found in the vast ocean of Tibetan medical knowledge. Needless to say, someone such as myself, with inferior knowledge and lack of experience, can misunderstand and make mistakes. Accordingly, I invite qualified scholars with knowledge and experience in Tibetan medicine to suggest any corrections to this compilation that they deem relevant.

From the 16th to the 25th days of the second month of the fire dog year 3924 (April 14 to 23, 2006), at Tashigar Norte, a seat of the Dzogchen Community in South America, I revised the text for the purpose of teaching interested students the material contained in this condensed manual of moxibustion. A preliminary set of the point drawings and the tables was prepared by my students Fabio Andrico, Alexey Polionov, and Elio Guarisco, to whom I extend my gratitude. My gratitude goes also to Tashigar Norte, which beautifully arranged all the necessary facilities.

A little more than a week before I was to begin to teach the moxibustion text, I noted some corrections and changes to the text were needed, and I added a few clarifications.

The editorial and layout work was completed between 2009 and 2011. Several revisions were made at this time; Tanita Ferrari created a new set of drawings with the assistance of Elio Guarisco and Alexey Polionov.

May this manual on the practice of moxibustion, which I have written with sincere intentions, bring great benefit to countless beings without distinction.

POINT
DRAWINGS

LIST OF PLATES

PLATE I.A
POINTS ALONG THE SPINE

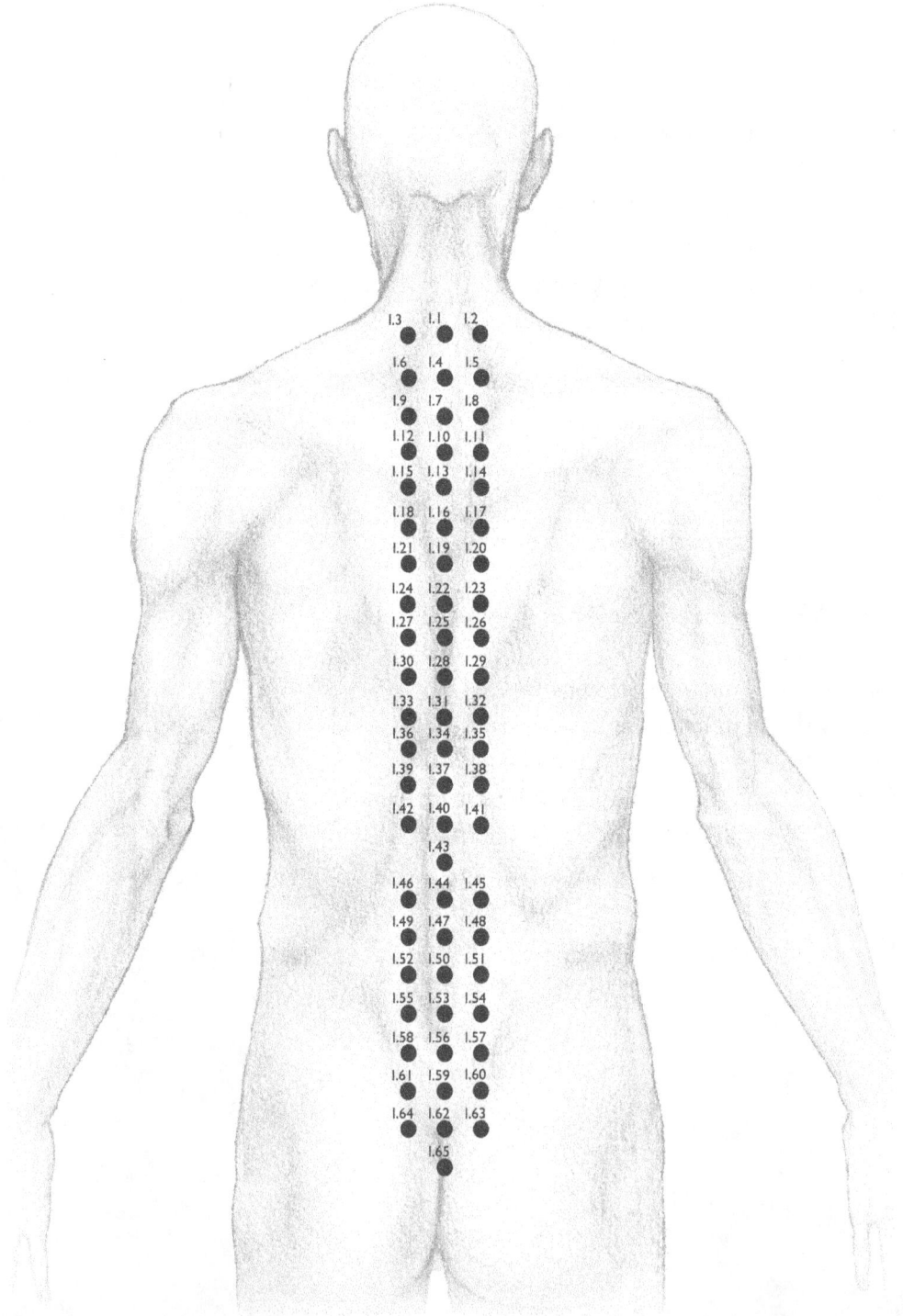

I.3 I.1 I.2
I.6 I.4 I.5
I.9 I.7 I.8
I.12 I.10 I.11
I.15 I.13 I.14
I.18 I.16 I.17
I.21 I.19 I.20
I.24 I.22 I.23
I.27 I.25 I.26
I.30 I.28 I.29
I.33 I.31 I.32
I.36 I.34 I.35
I.39 I.37 I.38
I.42 I.40 I.41
I.43
I.46 I.44 I.45
I.49 I.47 I.48
I.52 I.50 I.51
I.55 I.53 I.54
I.58 I.56 I.57
I.61 I.59 I.60
I.64 I.62 I.63
I.65

PLATE I.B
UPPER POINTS ALONG THE SPINE

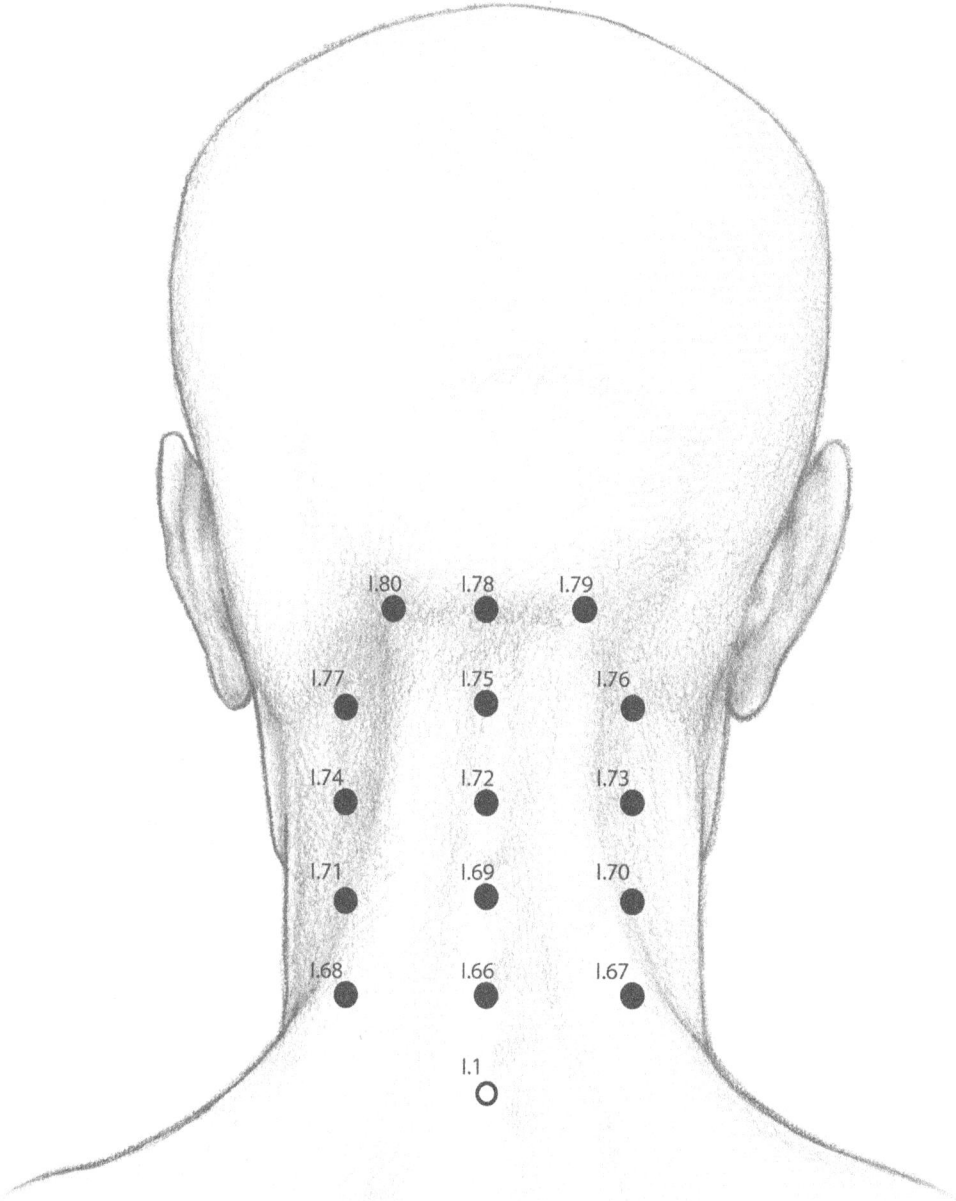

I.80   I.78   I.79

I.77   I.75   I.76

I.74   I.72   I.73

I.71   I.69   I.70

I.68   I.66   I.67

I.1

PLATE II.A
UPPER POINTS ON THE LATERAL BACK

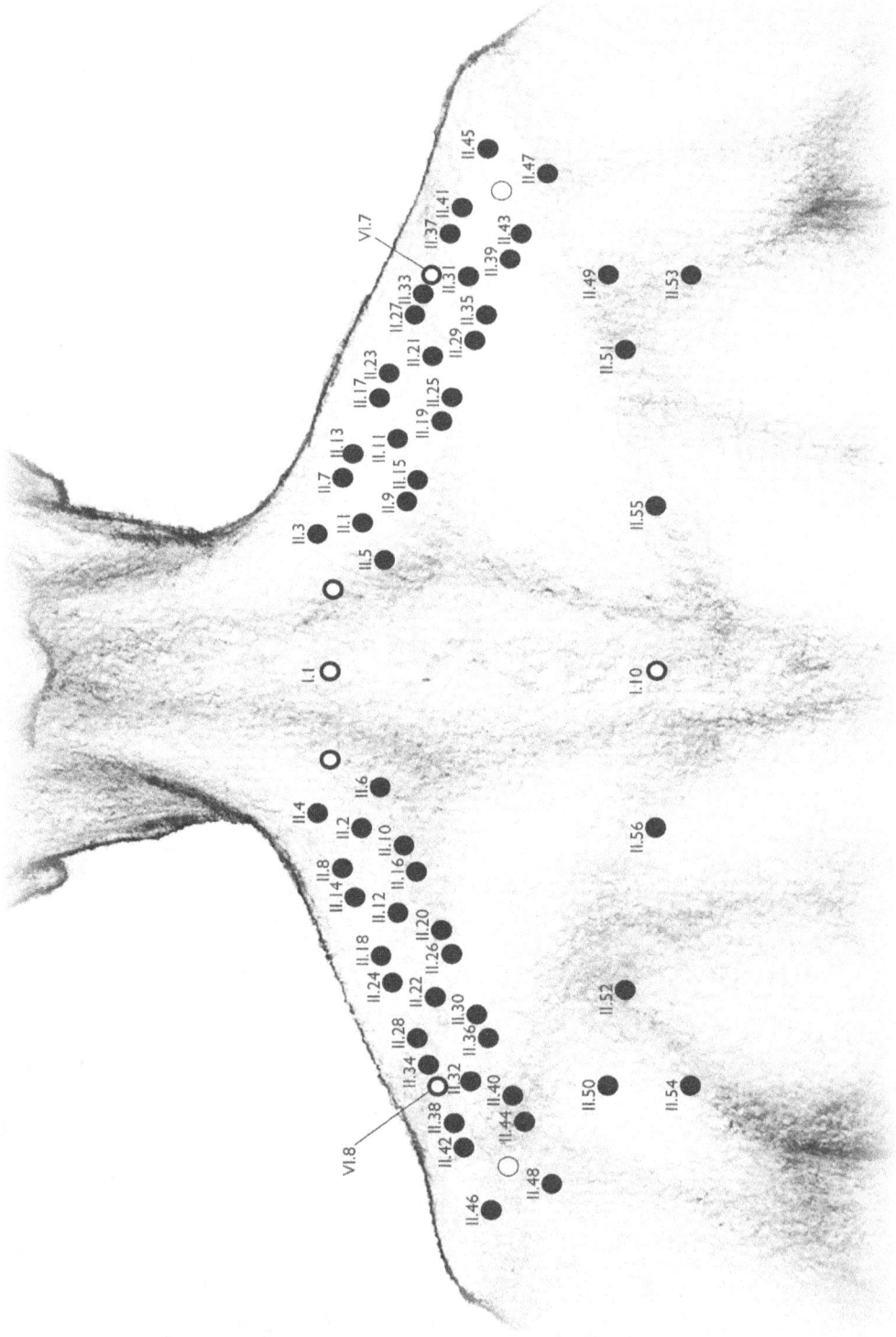

PLATE II.B
POINTS ON THE LATERAL BACK

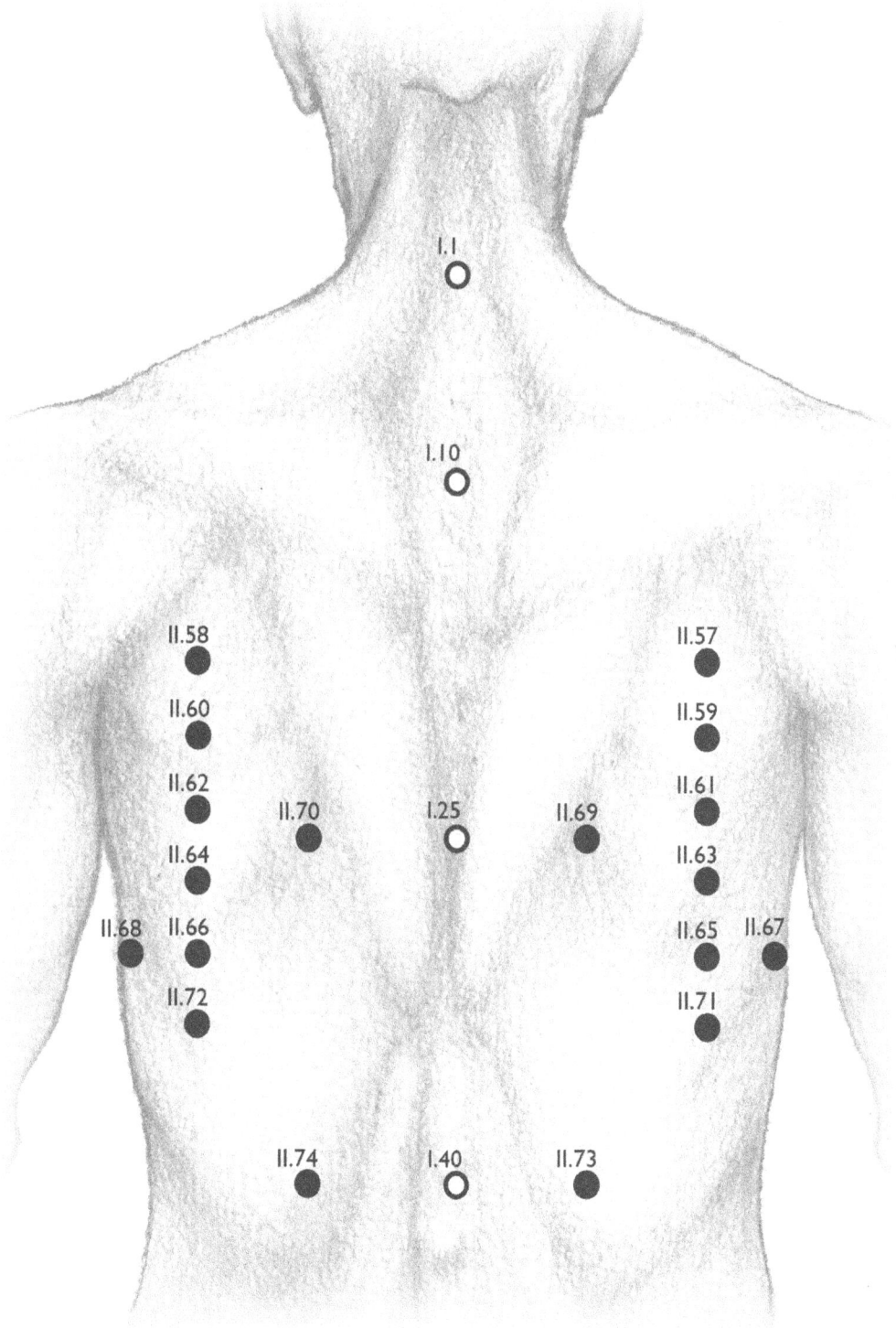

I.1
○

I.10
○

II.58
●

II.57
●

II.60
●

II.59
●

II.62
●

II.70
●

I.25
○

II.69
●

II.61
●

II.64
●

II.63
●

II.68   II.66
●   ●

II.65   II.67
●   ●

II.72
●

II.71
●

II.74
●

I.40
○

II.73
●

Plate III.a
Upper Points on the Central Front of the Torso

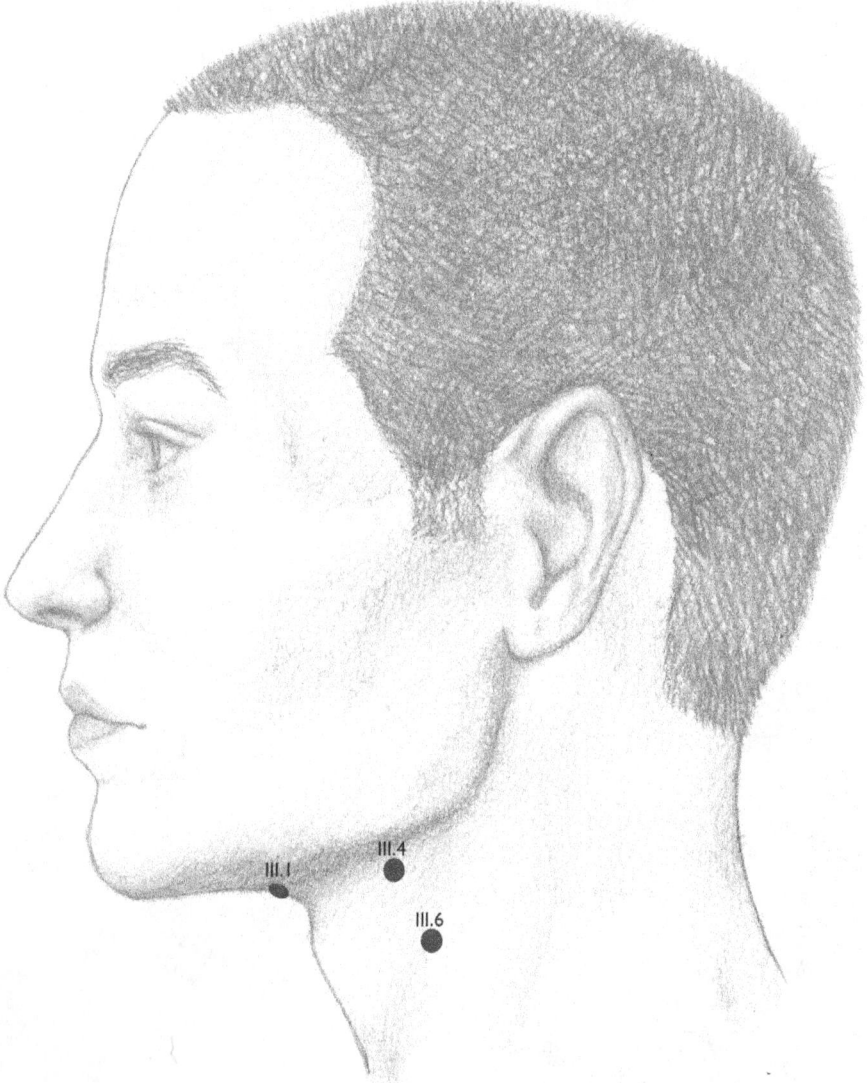

III.1

III.4

III.6

PLATE III.b
POINTS ON THE CENTRAL FRONT OF THE TORSO

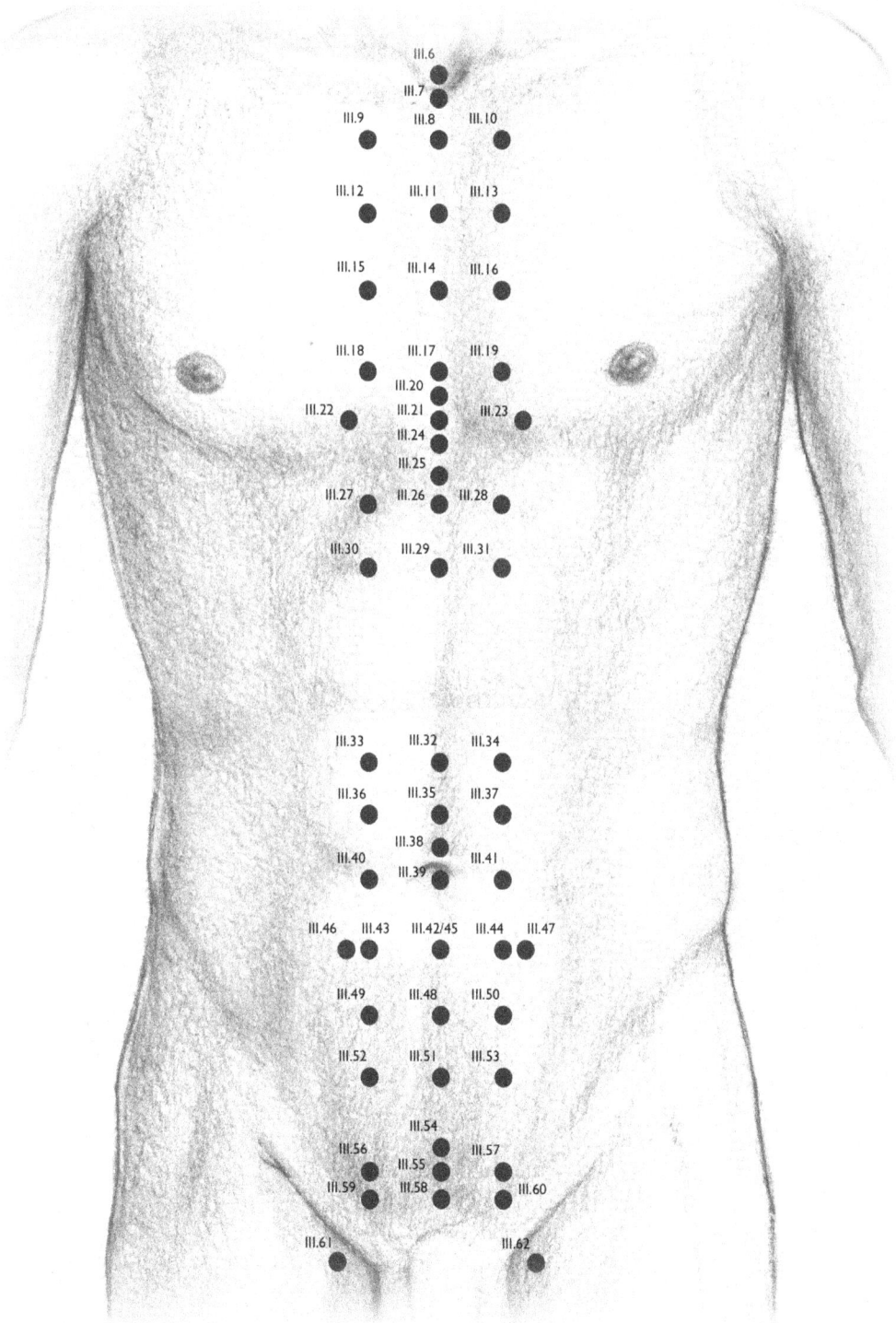

III.6
III.7
III.9   III.8   III.10
III.12   III.11   III.13
III.15   III.14   III.16
III.18   III.17   III.19
         III.20
III.22   III.21   III.23
         III.24
         III.25
III.27   III.26   III.28
III.30   III.29   III.31

III.33   III.32   III.34
III.36   III.35   III.37
         III.38
III.40   III.39   III.41
III.46 III.43 III.42/45 III.44 III.47
III.49   III.48   III.50
III.52   III.51   III.53
         III.54
III.56   III.55   III.57
III.59   III.58   III.60
III.61   III.62

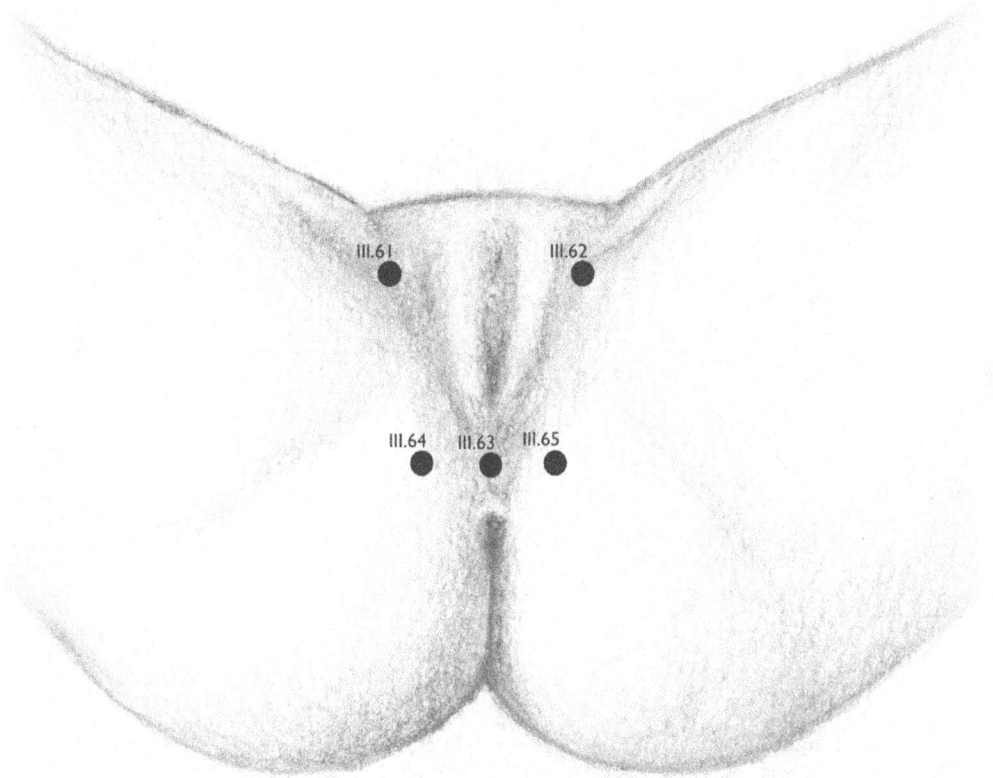

PLATE III.C
LOWER POINTS ON THE FRONT OF THE TORSO

PLATE IV
POINTS ON THE LATERAL FRONT OF THE TORSO

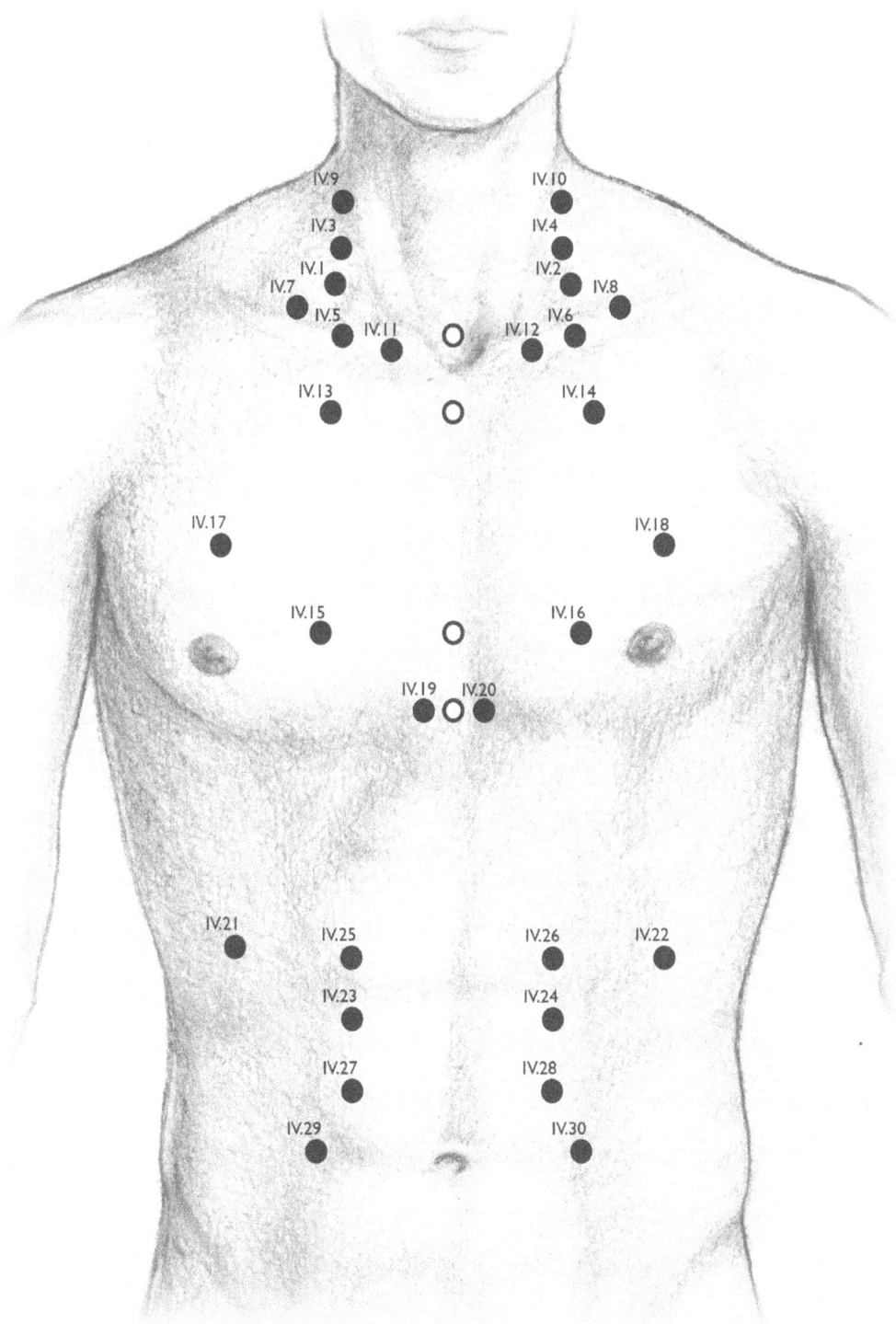

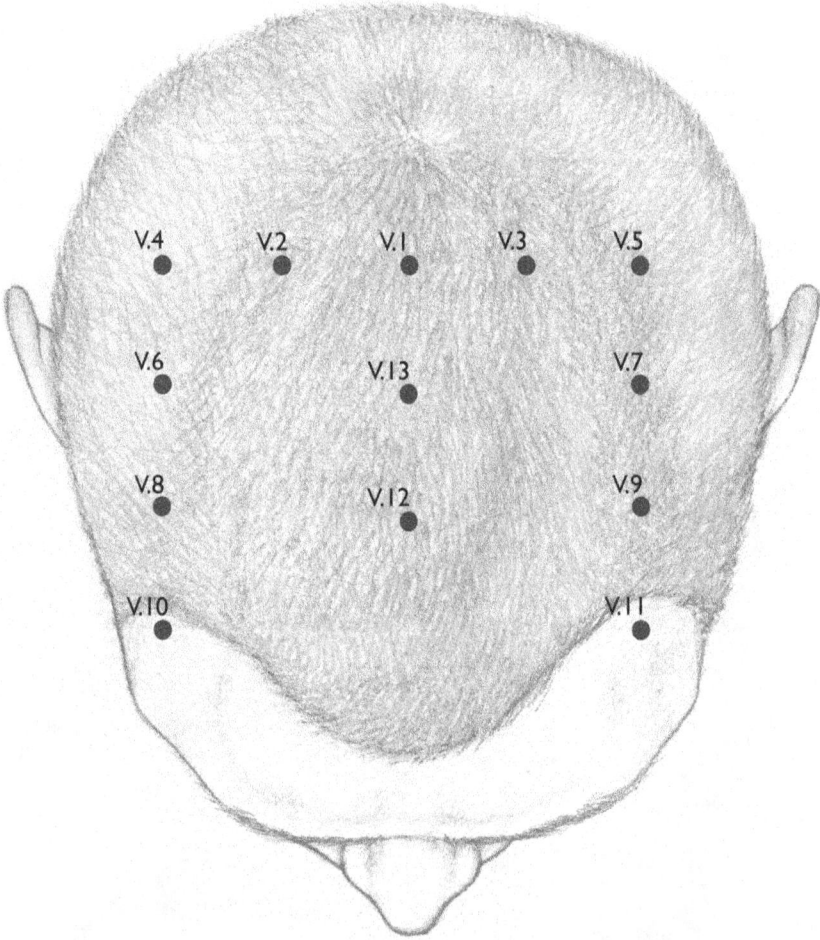

PLATE V.A
POINTS ON THE HEAD, TOP

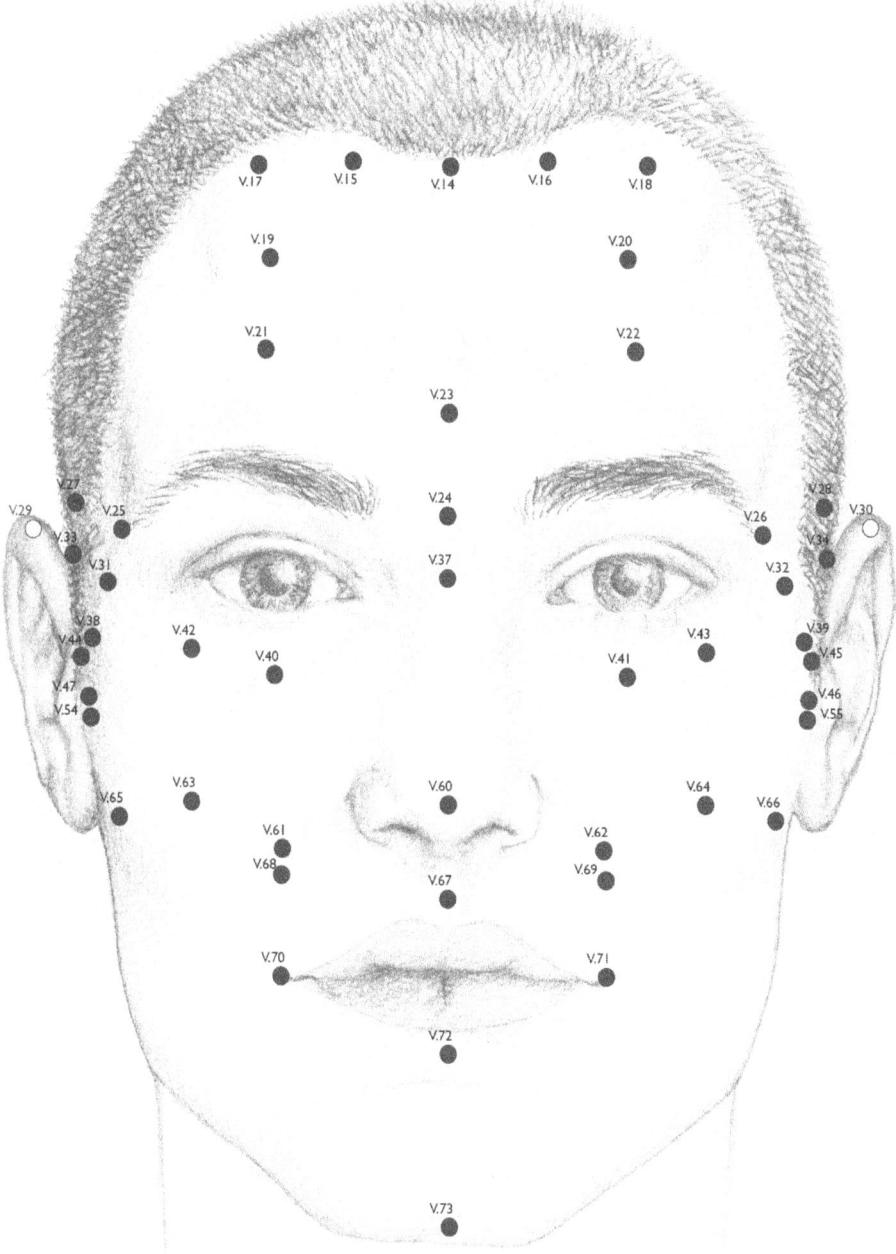

PLATE V.B
POINTS ON THE HEAD, FRONT

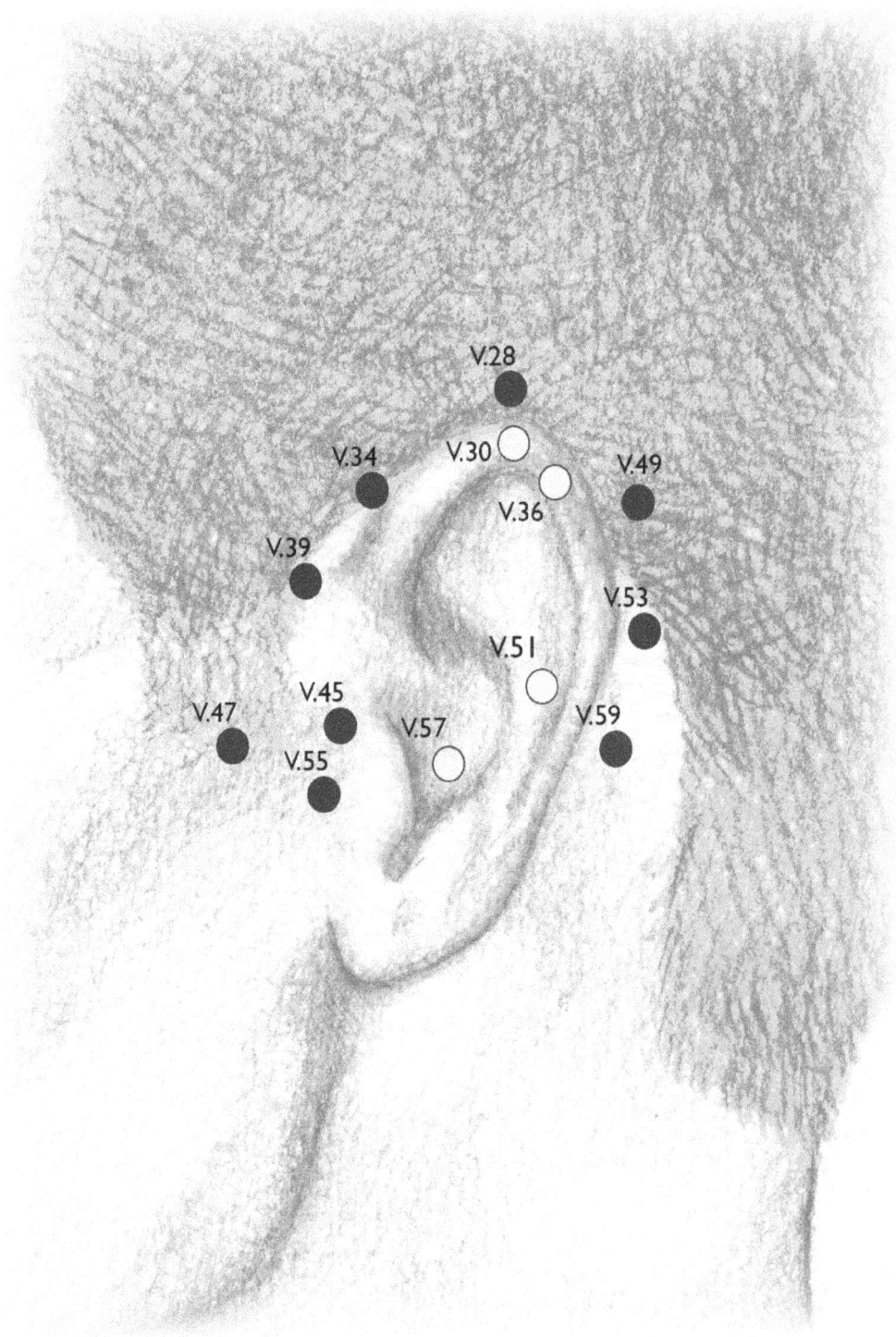

PLATE V.C
POINTS ON THE HEAD, SIDE

V.28

V.34 V.30 V.49

V.36

V.39

V.53

V.51

V.45 V.59

V.47 V.57

V.55

PLATE V.D
POINTS ON THE HEAD, BACK

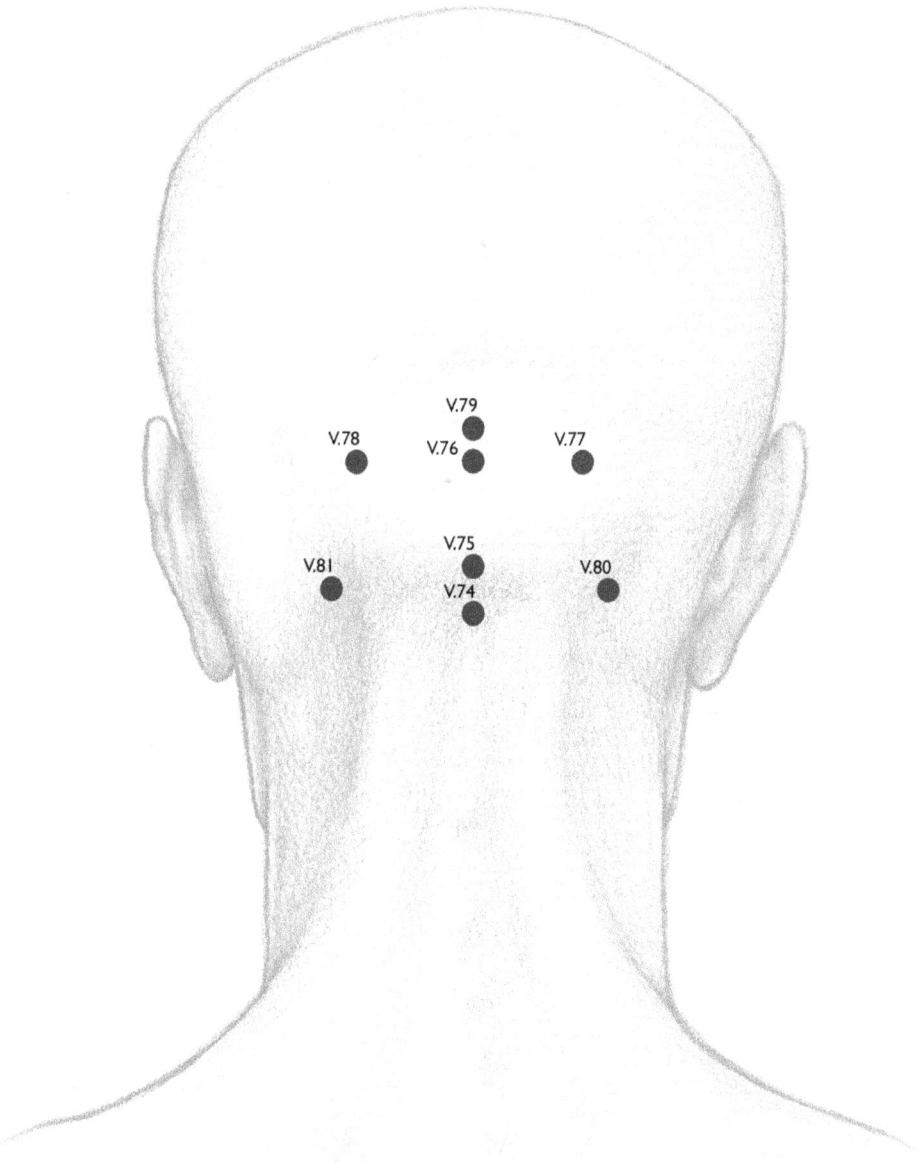

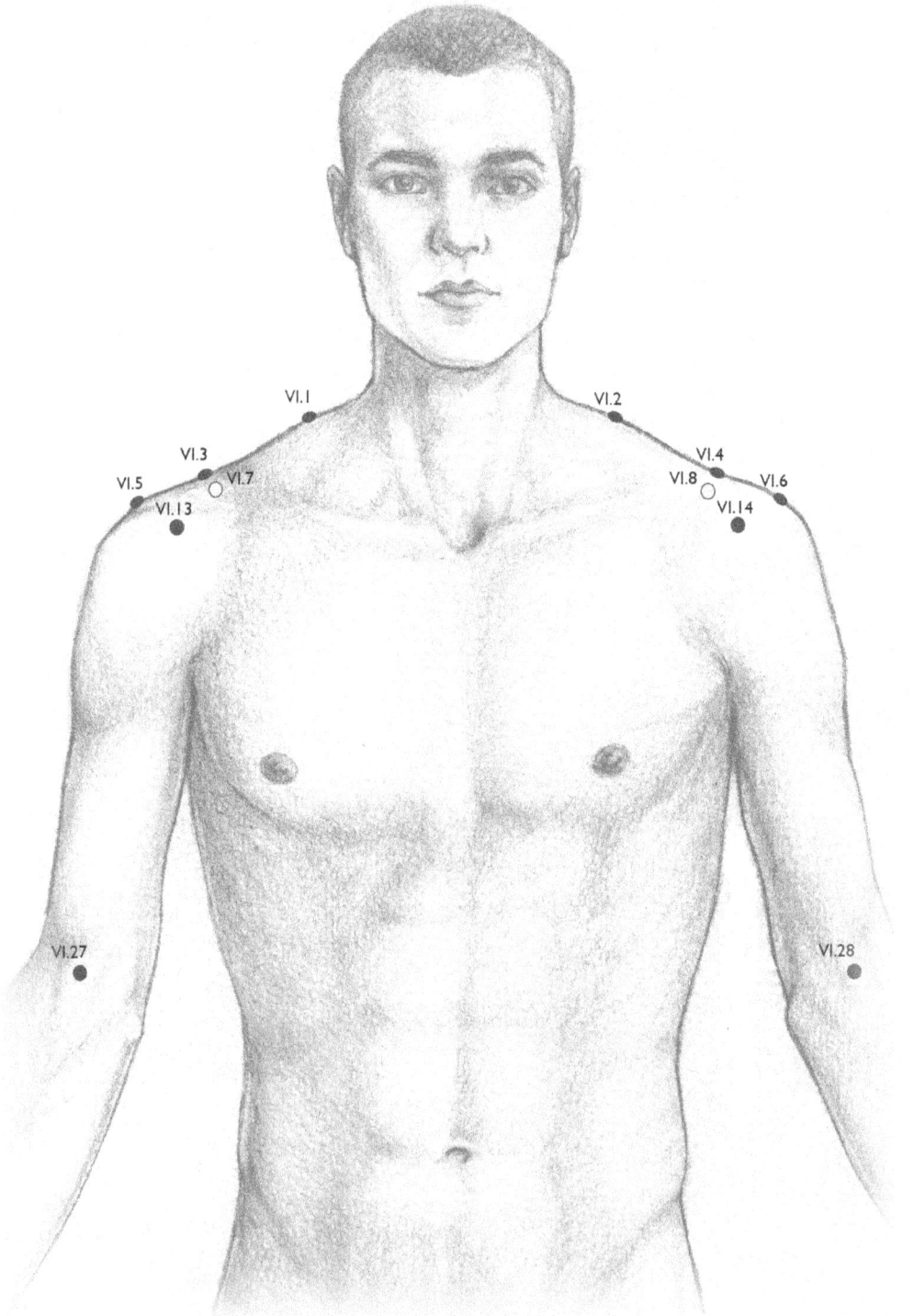

PLATE VI.A
UPPER POINTS ON THE ARMS

VI.1
VI.2
VI.3
VI.4
VI.5   VI.7   VI.8   VI.6
VI.13   VI.14
VI.27   VI.28

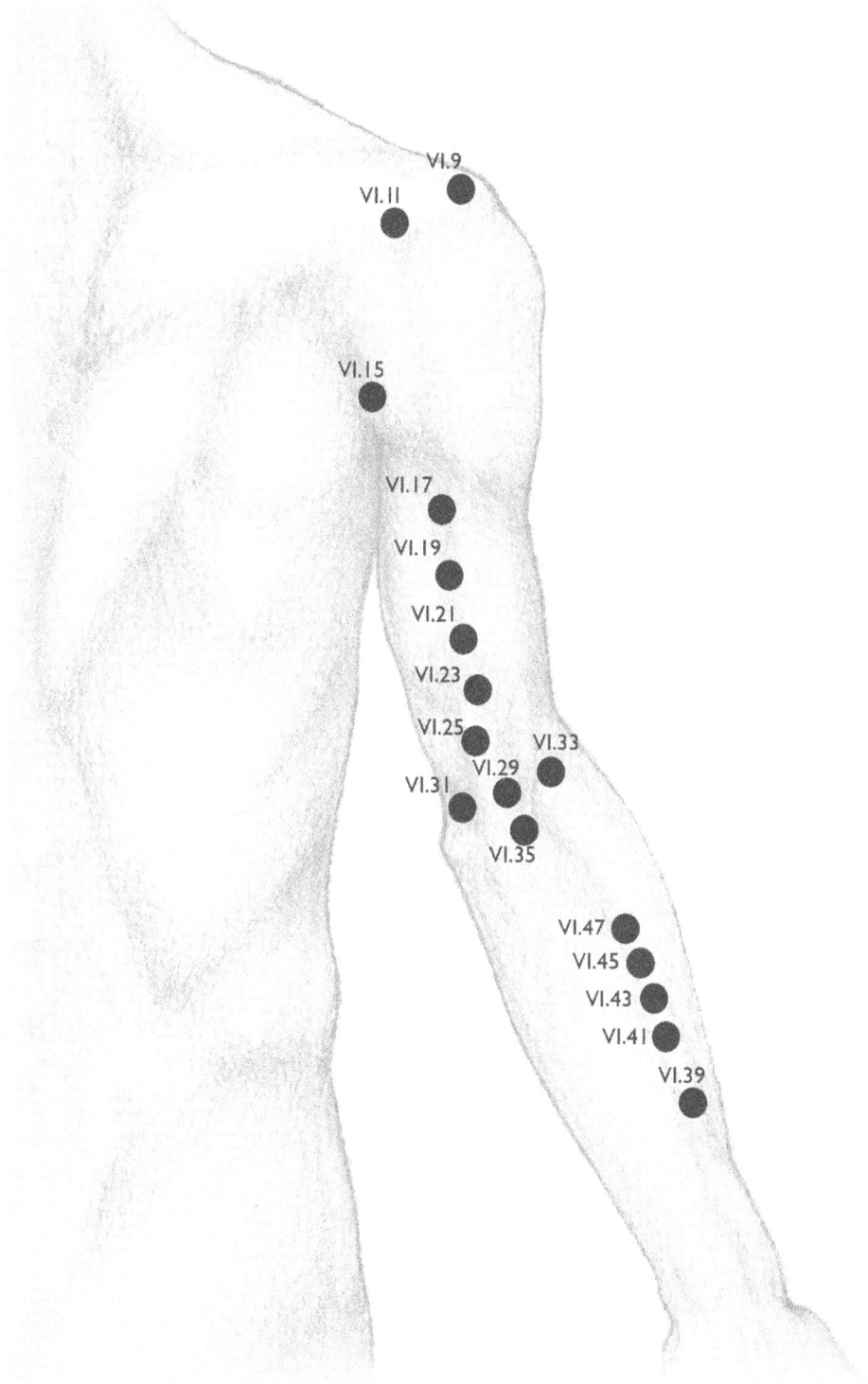

PLATE VI.B
BACK POINTS ON THE ARMS

VI.9

VI.11

VI.15

VI.17

VI.19

VI.21

VI.23

VI.25

VI.33

VI.29

VI.31

VI.35

VI.47

VI.45

VI.43

VI.41

VI.39

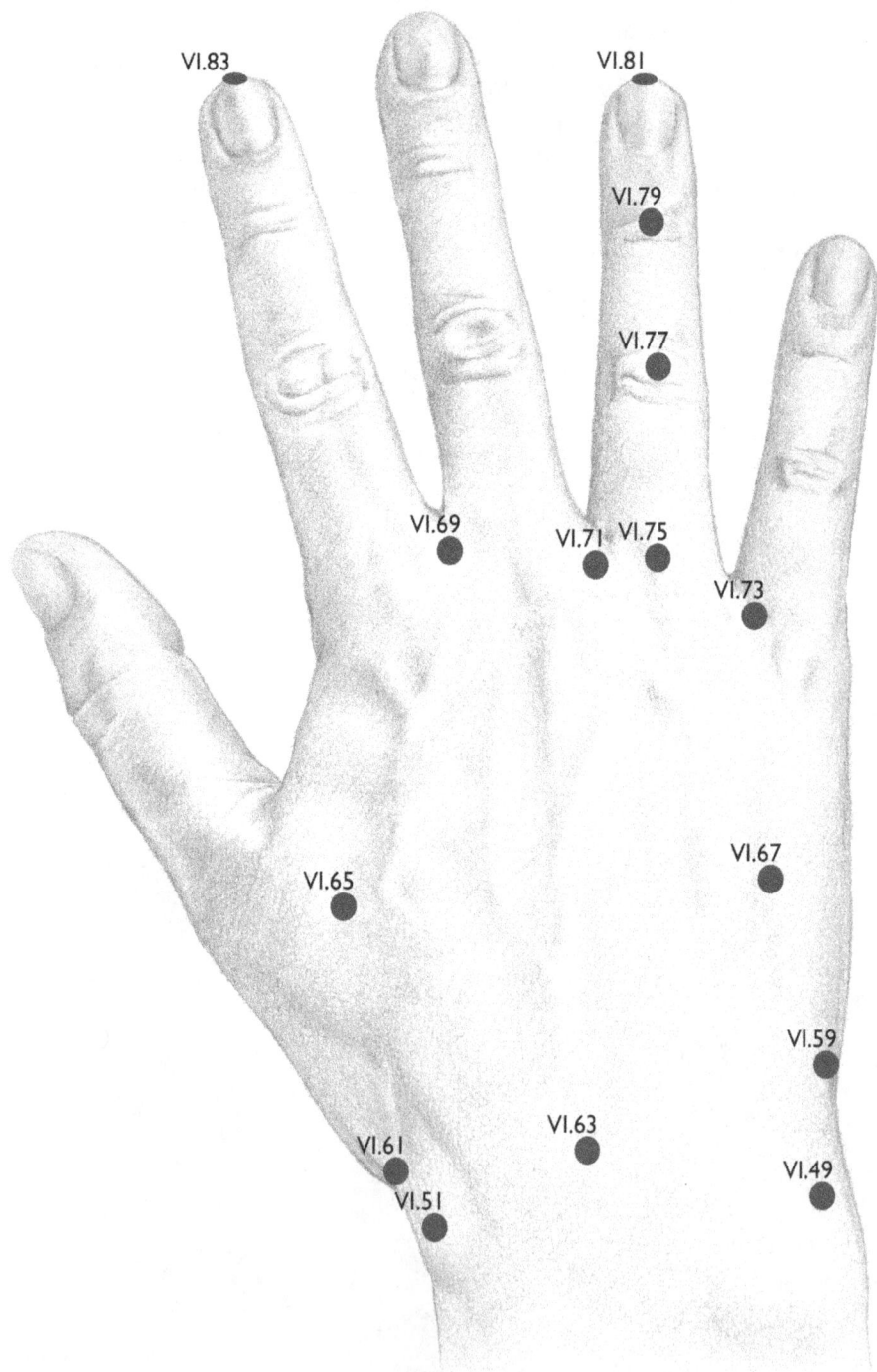

PLATE VI.c
POINTS ON THE ARMS, BACK OF THE HAND

VI.83
VI.81
VI.79
VI.77
VI.69
VI.71 VI.75
VI.73
VI.67
VI.65
VI.59
VI.63
VI.61
VI.49
VI.51

PLATE VI.d
POINTS ON THE ARMS, FRONT OF THE HAND AND
LOWER ARM

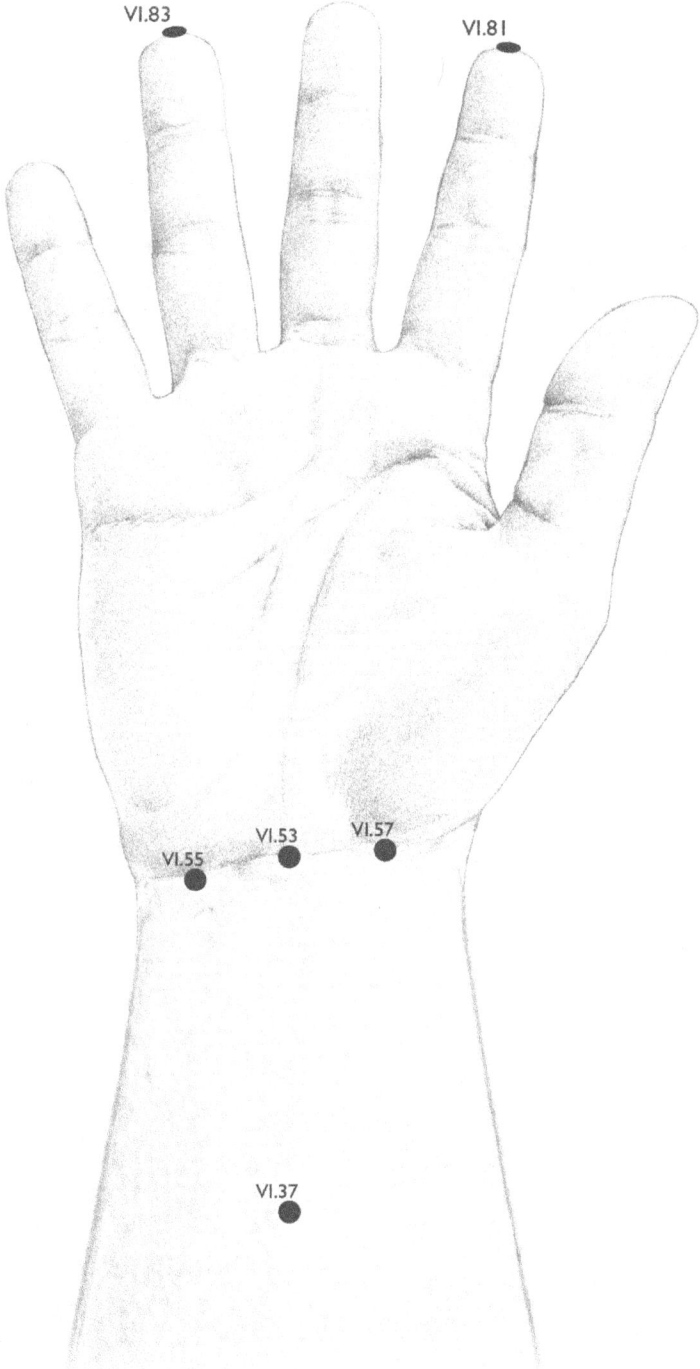

VI.83

VI.81

VI.57

VI.53

VI.55

VI.37

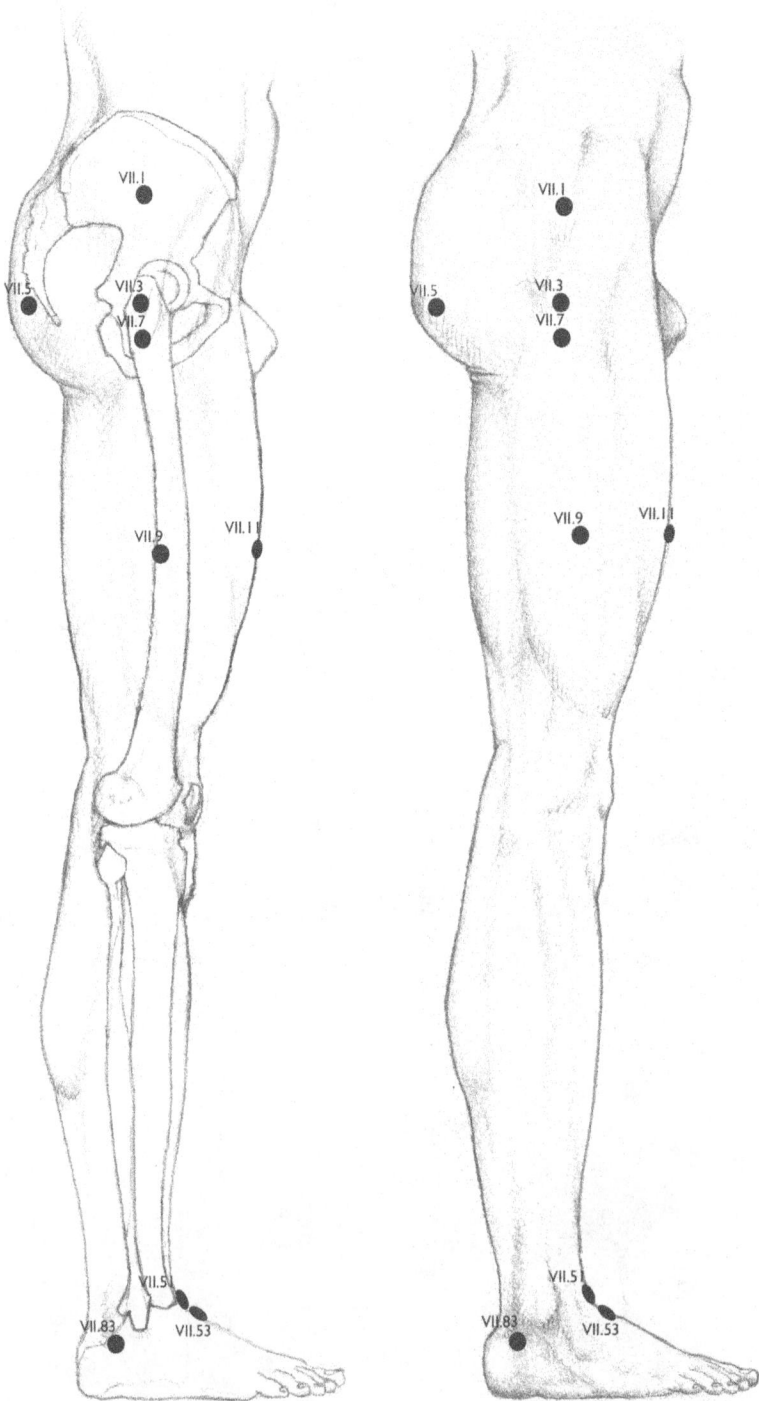

PLATE VII.a
POINTS ON THE LEGS, SIDE

VII.1

VII.5   VII.3
         VII.7

VII.9   VII.11

VII.1

VII.5   VII.3
         VII.7

VII.9   VII.11

VII.51
VII.83   VII.53

VII.51
VII.83   VII.53

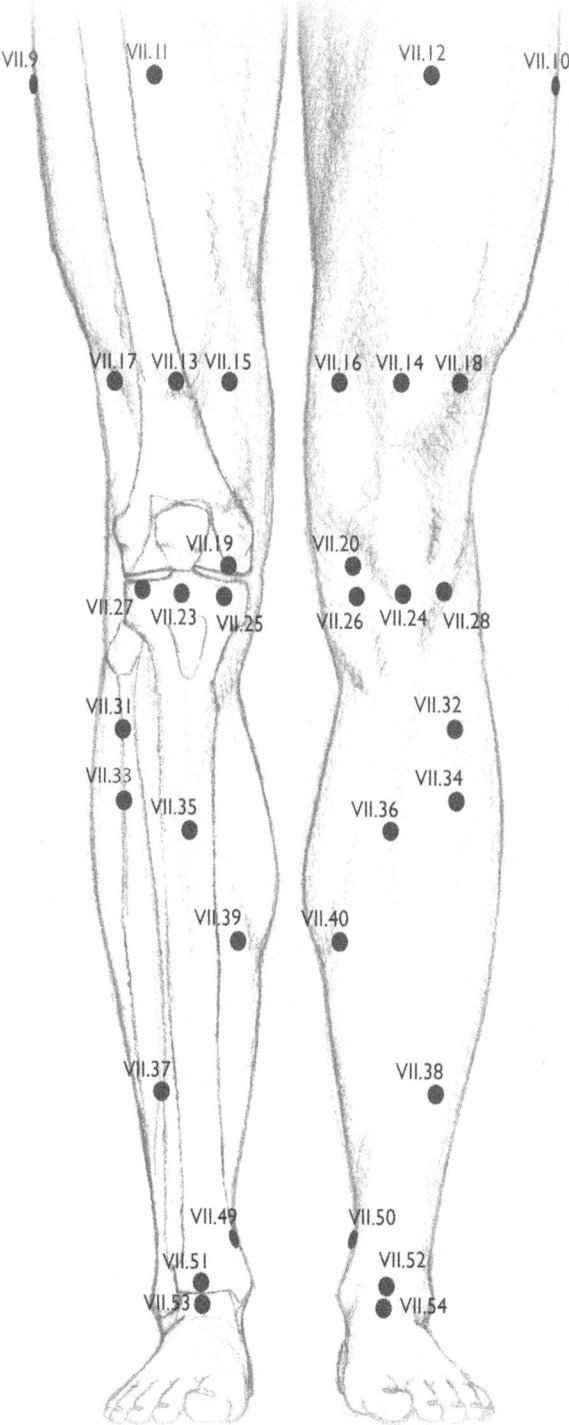

PLATE VII.b
POINTS ON THE LEGS, FRONT

VII.9 VII.11 VII.12 VII.10

VII.17 VII.13 VII.15 VII.16 VII.14 VII.18

VII.19 VII.20

VII.27 VII.23 VII.25 VII.26 VII.24 VII.28

VII.31 VII.32

VII.33 VII.34

VII.35 VII.36

VII.39 VII.40

VII.37 VII.38

VII.49 VII.50

VII.51 VII.52

VII.53 VII.54

PLATE VII.c
POINTS ON THE LEGS, BACK

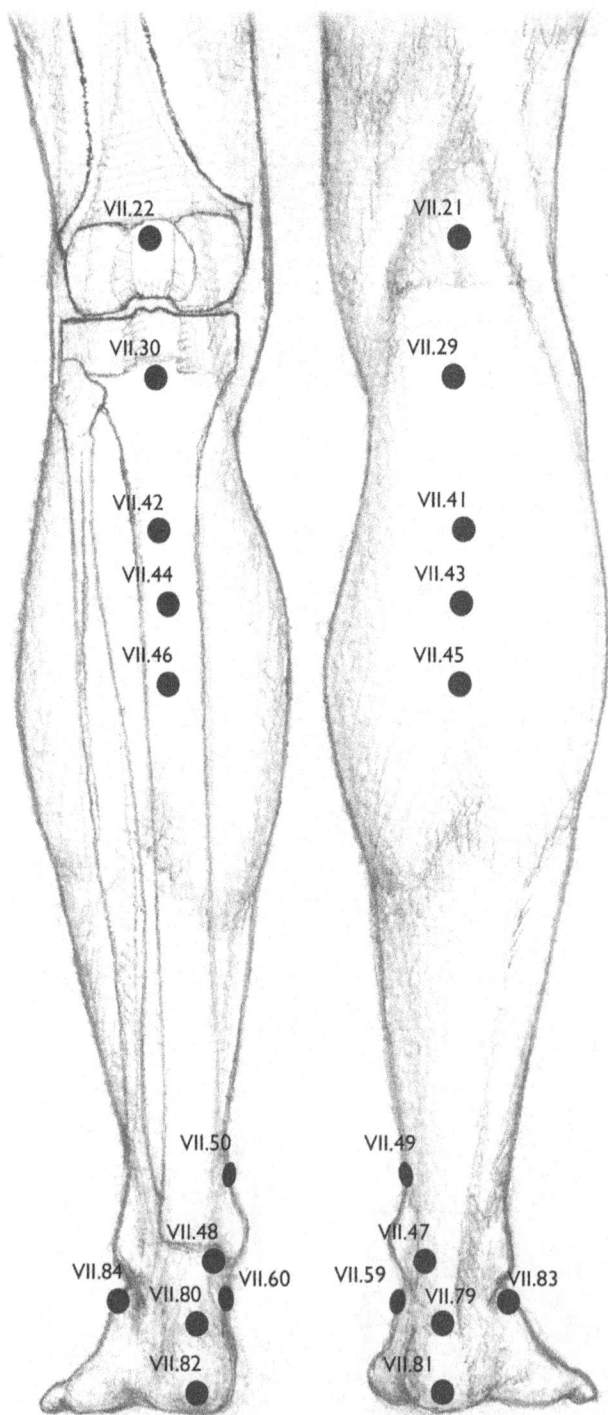

VII.22

VII.21

VII.30

VII.29

VII.42

VII.41

VII.44

VII.43

VII.46

VII.45

VII.50

VII.49

VII.48

VII.47

VII.84

VII.59

VII.83

VII.80

VII.60

VII.79

VII.82

VII.81

PLATE VII.d
POINTS ON THE LEGS, OUTER FOOT

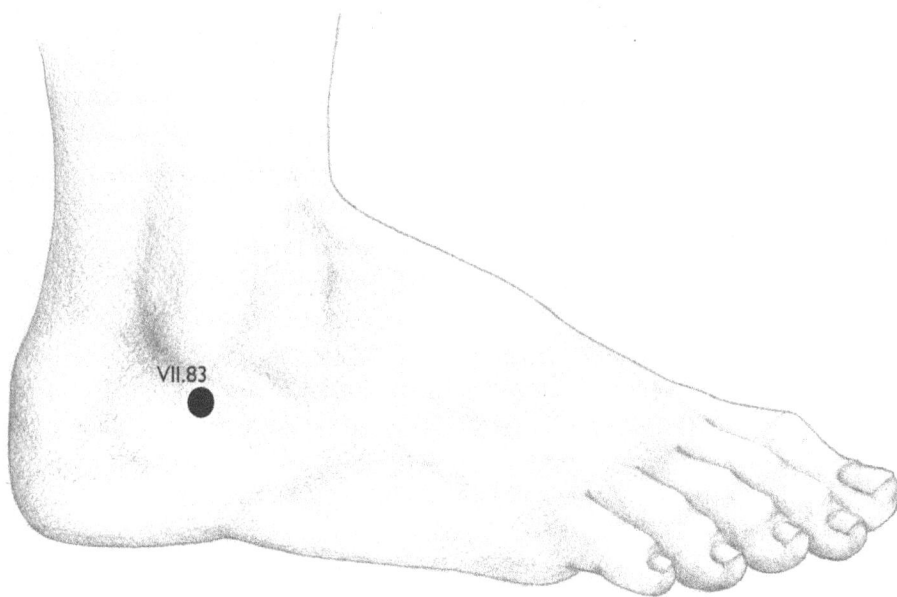

PLATE VII.e
POINTS ON THE LEGS, INNER FOOT

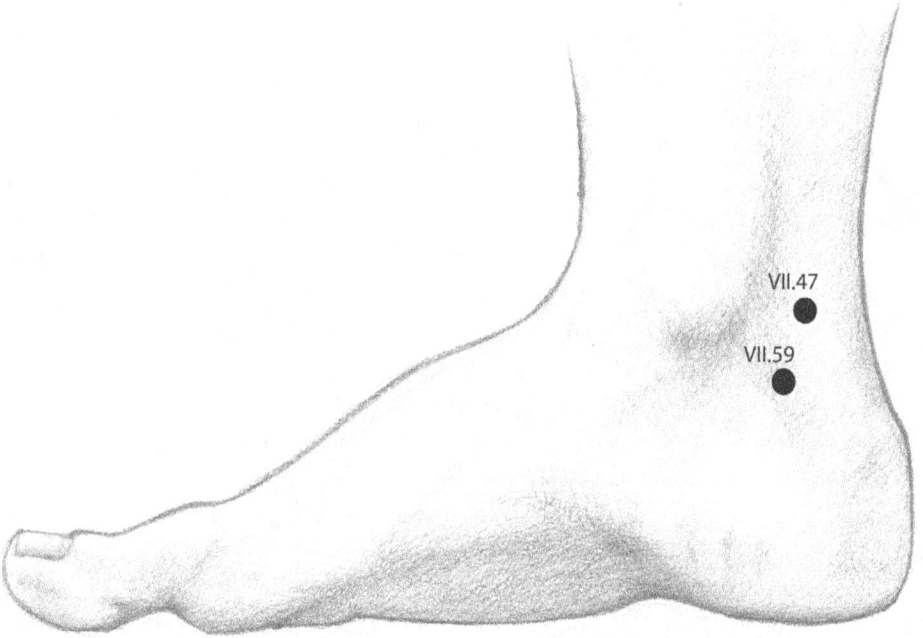

PLATE VII.f
POINTS ON THE LEGS, BACK OF THE FOOT

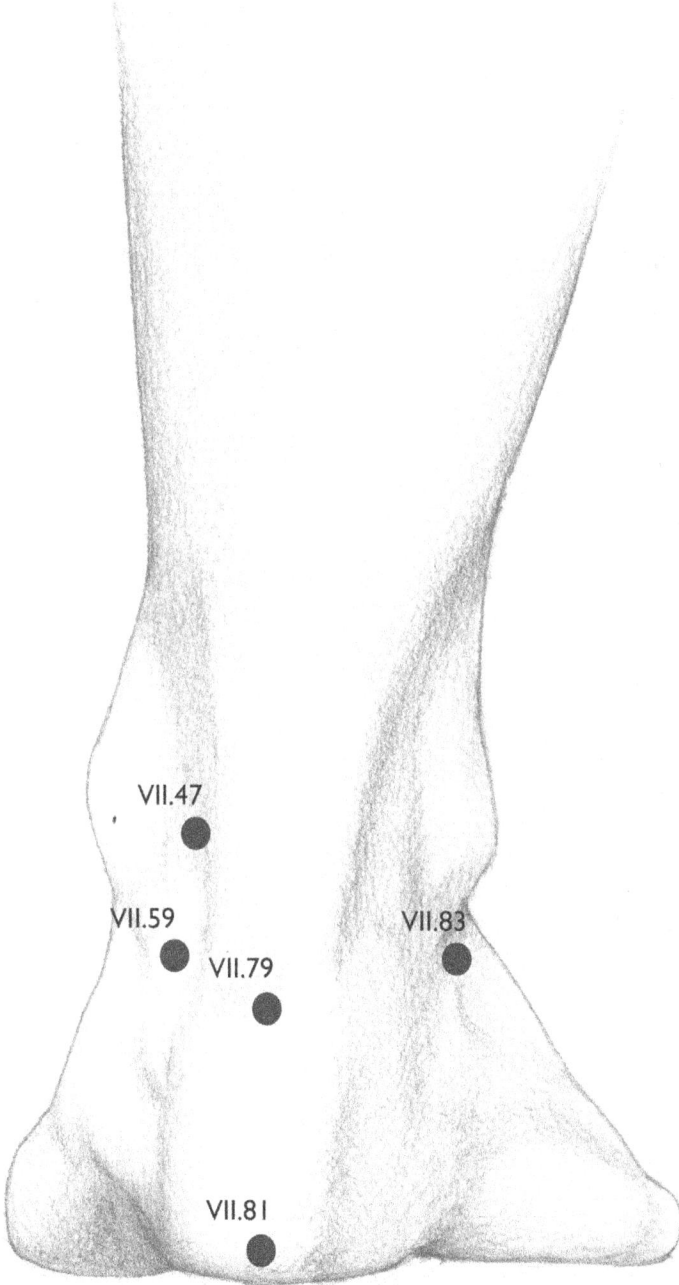

VII.47

VII.59

VII.83

VII.79

VII.81

PLATE VII.g
POINTS ON THE LEGS, TOP OF THE FOOT

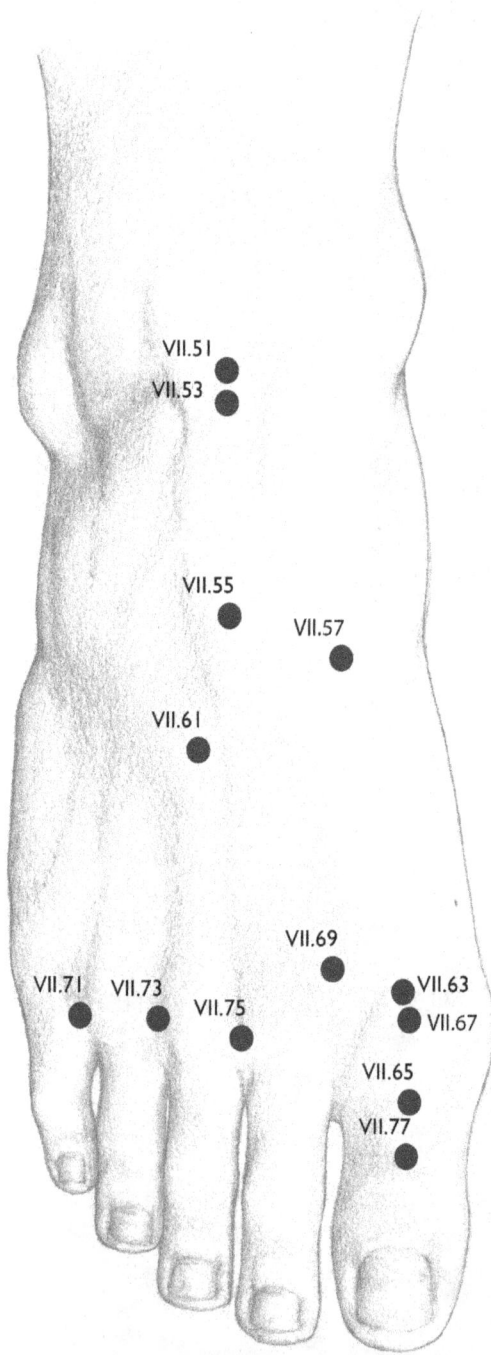

VII.51

VII.53

VII.55

VII.57

VII.61

VII.69

VII.71 VII.73 VII.75

VII.63

VII.67

VII.65

VII.77

PLATE VII.h
POINTS ON THE LEGS, SOLE OF THE FOOT

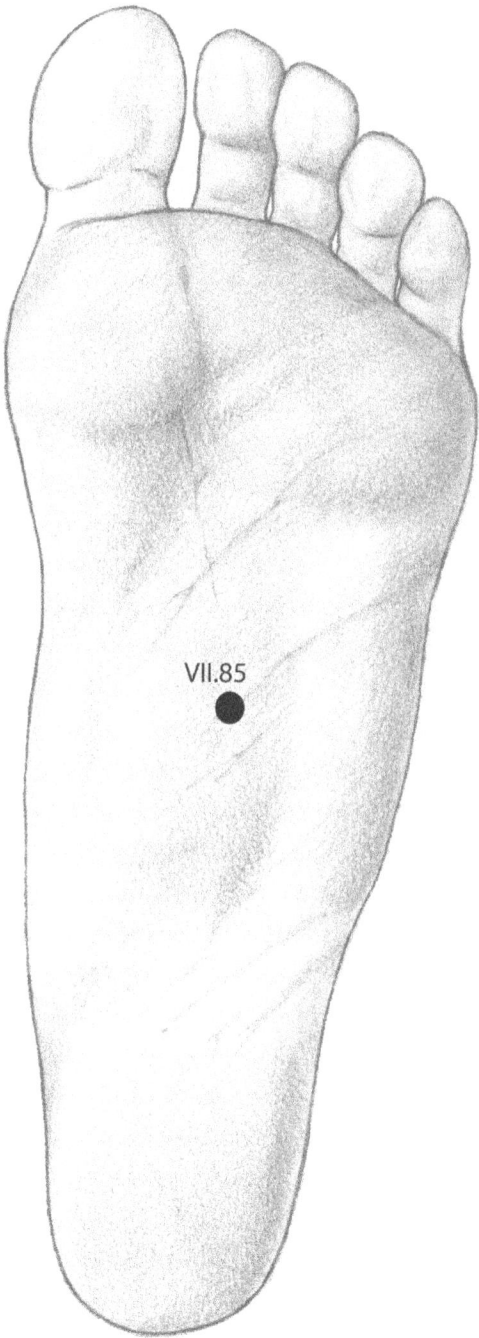

VII.85

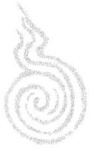

Appendix A

ASTROLOGICAL FACTORS

According to Tibetan medicine, strong external therapies are contraindicated under certain astrological conditions.[1] Astrological manuals specify three different factors that need to be considered when weighing the appropriateness of the timing of external therapies. Each will be explained in greater detail below. Specifically, Tibetan elemental astrology states that treatment should be avoided

- when the position of the protective energy of the individual is in the area to be treated;[2]
- at the time of day when the astrological influence of *viṣṭi*[3] is present;
- on the days during which *Nāga Kulika*[4] exerts its influence.

It is important to emphasize that these factors are primarily relevant for external therapies and procedures that can be regarded as invasive. In the case of moxibustion, apart from the direct application of moxa, and in particular treatments involving the cauterization of the skin, none of the other forms of treatment pose a significant risk for the patient, even if performed without due consideration given to the position of the individual's protective energy and the other factors discussed in this appendix. Still, direct experience has shown that therapies of any type, including moxa, are more effective if the treatment is applied in a location as far as possible from the place where the protective energy temporarily resides. The same applies analogously to the other astrological factors referred to here.[5]

HOW TO CALCULATE ASTROLOGICAL FACTORS INFLUENCING TREATMENT

I. PROTECTIVE ENERGY (LA)
Several factors need to be taken into consideration to identify when an individual's protective energy is located in a particular position.

The Significance of the Position of the Protective Energy

La, or protective energy, refers to the power of the elements that are the base of the life force of an individual. Should the protective energy, the base of the life force, decline, disperse, or separate from the elements of the body of an individual, various types of damage to the life force and body of the individual could result. Moreover, a variety of obstacles could also occur, such as the weakening and decline of the individual's capacity and good fortune. It is therefore of utmost importance that an individual's protective energy be in good condition throughout his or her life.

Accordingly, it is harmful to apply strong external therapies on specific areas when the protective energy is transiting there, especially treatments such as a direct application of moxa involving cauterization of the skin. Indeed, in some cases, this can be very dangerous.

These risks are explained in detail in numerous astrological texts:[6]

- When the therapy is applied on the location where the protective energy resides together with the patient's Deity of Life, it can become a secondary cause for the death of that patient.
- When the therapy is applied on the location where the protective energy resides together with the patient's Deity of the Body, it can become a secondary cause for a serious injury or paralysis.
- When the therapy is applied on the location where the protective energy resides together with the Deity of Capacity, it can become a secondary cause for the decline of the patient's capacity.
- When the therapy is applied on the location where the protective energy resides together with the Deity of Fortune, it can become a secondary cause for a short lifespan and the decline of the patient's good fortune.
- When the therapy is applied on the location where the protective energy resides together with the Deity of Birth, it can become a secondary cause for weakening the patient's strength and radiance.

SPECIFIC POSITIONS OF THE PROTECTIVE ENERGY

Protective energy has five different positions:[7]

i) *Position of the protective energy in relation to the year*
ii) *Position of the protective energy in relation to the days of the lunar month*
iii) *Position of the protective energy in relation to the days of the week*
iv) *Position of the protective energy in relation to different periods of the days of the lunar month*
v) *Position of the protective energy in relation to critical periods of the day*

i) Position of the protective energy in relation to the year

The eight trigrams indicate in which part of an individual's body the protective energy is located in a given year. Performing a strong external therapy such as moxa on the body part with which the trigram of the year is associated is to be avoided as it can become a secondary cause for the patient's illness to linger for long time and for additional illnesses to arise. It is therefore extremely important to understand the need to carefully refrain from applying all types of major external therapies on the area corresponding with the yearly position of the protective energy.

A complete cycle of trigrams unfolds in two cycles of sixty years, as shown in the following table.[8]

The 120-Year Cycle for the Trigram of the Year

	Animal	Mouse	Ox	Tiger	Hare	Dragon	Snake	Horse	Sheep	Monkey	Bird	Dog	Boar
1st Cycle	ELEMENT	Wood	Wood	Fire	Fire	Earth	Earth	Metal	Metal	Water	Water	Wood	Wood
	TRIGRAM	li	khon	dwa	khen	kham	gin	zin	zon	li	khon	dwa	khen
	ELEMENT	Fire	Fire	Earth	Earth	Metal	Metal	Water	Water	Wood	Wood	Fire	Fire
	TRIGRAM	kham	gin	zin	zon	li	khon	dwa	khen	kham	gin	zin	zon
	ELEMENT	Earth	Earth	Metal	Metal	Water	Water	Wood	Wood	Fire	Fire	Earth	Earth
	TRIGRAM	li	khon	dwa	khen	kham	gin	zin	zon	li	khon	dwa	khen
	ELEMENT	Metal	Metal	Water	Water	Wood	Wood	Fire	Fire	Earth	Earth	Metal	Metal
	TRIGRAM	kham	gin	zin	zon	li	khon	dwa	khen	kham	gin	zin	zon
	ELEMENT	Water	Water	Wood	Wood	Fire	Fire	Earth	Earth	Metal	Metal	Water	Water
	TRIGRAM	li	khon	dwa	khen	kham	gin	zin	zon	li	khon	dwa	khen
2nd Cycle	ELEMENT	Wood	Wood	Fire	Fire	Earth	Earth	Metal	Metal	Water	Water	Wood	Wood
	TRIGRAM	kham	gin	zin	zon	li	khon	dwa	khen	kham	gin	zin	zon
	ELEMENT	Fire	Fire	Earth	Earth	Metal	Metal	Water	Water	Wood	Wood	Fire	Fire
	TRIGRAM	li	khon	dwa	khen	kham	gin	zin	zon	li	khon	dwa	khen
	ELEMENT	Earth	Earth	Metal	Metal	Water	Water	Wood	Wood	Fire	Fire	Earth	Earth
	TRIGRAM	kham	gin	zin	zon	li	khon	dwa	khen	kham	gin	zin	zon
	ELEMENT	Metal	Metal	Water	Water	Wood	Wood	Fire	Fire	Earth	Earth	Metal	Metal
	TRIGRAM	li	khon	dwa	khen	kham	gin	zin	zon	li	khon	dwa	khen
	ELEMENT	Water	Water	Wood	Wood	Fire	Fire	Earth	Earth	Metal	Metal	Water	Water
	TRIGRAM	kham	gin	zin	zon	li	khon	dwa	khen	kham	gin	zin	zon

▮ Wood[9]   ▲ Fire   ■ Earth   ⌒ Metal   ● Water

In Tibetan astrology, in addition to the eight trigrams, which are numbered in forward order (one, two, three... seven, eight), there are also nine *mewas* (*sme ba*), or numbers, which are numbered in reverse order (one, nine, eight... three, two). Since this ancient system of calculating the trigrams in the forward order and the *mewas* in the reverse order was prevalent in Shang Shung and Tibet, we have followed the same approach.

A 180-year cycle or *mekhor*[10] is comprised of three cycles of sixty years: the first, middle, and last sixty-year cycle.[11] Our present time falls within the last sixty-year cycle of the twenty-second 180-year cycle,[12] and within the second sixty years in the 120-cycle of trigrams.[13] Taking the metal dragon year that began on February 5, 2000, as an example, we can understand immediately that the trigram for that year was *kham*, the fifth trigram, by locating the metal dragon in the second cycle on the trigram chart.

Position of the Protective Energy in Relation to the Trigrams

Trigram	Location of the Protective Energy
li (1)	Head
khon (2)	Left hand
dwa (3)	Left side of the torso
khen (4)	Left foot
kham (5)	Genitals
gin (6)	Right foot
zin (7)	Right side of the torso
zon (8)	Right hand

As explained above, it is very important to avoid applying major kinds of external therapies on the locations where an individual's protective energy is dwelling in relation to the eight trigrams.[14]

ii) Position of the protective energy in relation to the days of the lunar month
According to experts in astrology, there are a number of different systems for identifying the position of the protective energy in relation to days of the lunar month, and it is difficult to rely on any one system alone.

The following table provides a general overview of the different methods for identifying the position of an individual's protective energy in relation to the days of the lunar month.

Principal Systems for Identifying the Protective Energy on the Days of the Lunar Month

Day of the Month	Zurkhar[15] System	Darmo[16] System	Mipham[17] System
1	Soles of the feet	Big toes	Big toes
2	Ankles	Ankles	Upper part of the feet
3	Thighs	Calves	Calf muscles
4	Waist	Medial thighs, from the knee up	Waist
5	Mouth	Back of the knees	Back of the knees
6	Chest	Lateral thighs	Lateral thighs
7	Back	Center of the chest	Hip sockets
8	Palms	Heart	Kidneys
9	Liver	Neck	Sides of the torso
10	Waist	Throat	Shoulders and shoulder blades
11	Nose	Tip of the nose	Forearms
12	Stomach	Forehead	Palm
13	Shoulder blades	Anterior fontanel	Front of the neck
14	Back of the hands	Tip of the ears	Temple
15	Entire body	Crown of the head, entire body	Shoulder blades
16	Neck	Occipital depression	Temple
17	Throat	Shoulder blades	Back of the neck
18	Stomach	Shoulders	Back of the hands
19	Ankles	Neck	Lateral forearms
20	Shanks	Elbows	Area of the shoulder blades
21	Big toes	Torso	Back of the torso
22	Left shoulder blade	Armpits	Area of the kidneys
23	Liver	Hands	Back of the hip sockets
24	Palms	Kidneys	Back of the thighs
25	Tongue	Hip sockets	Back of the knees
26	Knees	Lower shanks	Knees
27	Knees	Genitals	Back of the calf muscles
28	Genitals	Shanks	Back of the ankle joints
29	Both eyes	Back	Shanks
30	Entire body	Entire body	Entire body

The above table illustrates where the protective energy resides on each day of each lunar month. This understanding is crucial because on each of the thirty days related to the phases of the moon, it is important to carefully avoid performing any major external therapy on the indicated locations.

iii) Position of the protective energy in relation to the days of the week

Another factor considered in Tibetan astrology is the place where the position of the protective energy of the individual falls in relation to a particular day of the week.

Generally speaking, three distinct systems of astrology arose in ancient Tibet: the system derived from the *Concise Tantra of Kalachakra,*[18] the system of the highly learned astrologer Phugpa Lhundrup Gyatso,[19] and the ancient system of rediscovered astrological texts known as the *Early Translation Treasure House of Existence.*[20] However, with regard to identifying the position of the protective energy in relation to the days of the week, these three systems share the same approach.

The table below provides a concise overview of the location of an individual's protective energy for each day of the week. It is important to avoid applying any kind of major external therapy on those locations at these times since it may damage the protective energy of an individual.

Position of the Protective Energy in Relation to the Day of the Week

Day of the Week[21]	Location of Protective Energy
Sunday (1)	Head
Monday (2)	Breast, armpit
Tuesday (3)	Lungs, liver
Wednesday (4)	Waist area
Thursday (5)	Kidneys, waist
Friday (6)	Spinal column
Saturday (0)	Basilic vein[22]

iv) Position of the protective energy in relation to periods of the days of the lunar month[23]

Each of the thirty days of the lunar month in any year consists of twelve periods:

- Daybreak, the Period of the Rabbit (5 a.m.-7 a.m.)
- Sunrise, the Period of the Dragon (7 a.m.-9 a.m.)
- Mid-morning, the Period of the Snake (9 a.m.-11 a.m.)
- Midday, the Period of the Horse (11 a.m.-1 p.m.)
- Early afternoon, the Period of the Sheep (1 p.m.-3 p.m.)
- Late afternoon, the Period of the Monkey (3 p.m.-5 p.m.)
- Sunset, the Period of the Bird (5 p.m.-7 p.m.)
- Early evening, the Period of the Dog (7 p.m.-9 p.m.)
- Late evening, the Period of the Boar (9 p.m.-11 p.m.)
- Midnight, the Period of the Mouse (11 p.m.-1 a.m.)

• After midnight, the Period of the Ox (I a.m.-3 a.m.)
• Pre-dawn, the Period of the Tiger (3 a.m.-5 a.m.)[24]

The following table illustrates how to identify in which part of the body the protective energy of an individual resides in relation to these twelve periods on a given day of the lunar month.[25] It is important to avoid applying any kind of major external therapy on the respective locations at these times since it may damage the protective energy of an individual.

Correspondences Between Days of the Lunar Month & Periods of the Day

Day of the Lunar Month	Period of the Day	Location of Protective Energy
I	Mid-morning (9 a.m.-II a.m.)	Soles of the feet
2	From sunrise to mid-morning (7 a.m.-II a.m.)	Calves
3	Mid-morning (9 a.m.-II a.m.)	Thighs
4	Daybreak (5 a.m.-7 a.m.)	Waist
5	Sunset (5 p.m.-7 p.m.)	Inside the mouth
6	Mid-morning (9 a.m.-II a.m.)	Palms
7	Pre-dawn (3 a.m.-5 a.m.)	Ankles
8	Midnight (II p.m.-I a.m.)	Inner elbows
9	Daybreak (5 a.m.-7 a.m.)	Genitals
10	Late evening (9 p.m.-II p.m.)	Waist
II	Sunrise (7 a.m.-9 a.m.)	Right and left ears
12	Sunrise (7 a.m.-9 a.m.)	Hairline
13	Sunset (5 p.m.-7 p.m.)	Teeth
14	Midnight (II p.m.-I a.m.)	Heart
15	Late afternoon (3 p.m.-5 p.m.)	Entire body
16	--[26]	Center of the chest
17	Late evening (9 p.m.-II p.m.)	Left side of the neck
18	Mid-morning (9 a.m.-II a.m.)	Stomach, inner thighs
19	Daybreak (5 a.m.-7 a.m.)	Right and left thighs
20	Midday (II a.m.-I p.m.)	Right and left shin bones
21	Mid-morning (9 a.m.-II a.m.)	Soles of the feet
22	Daybreak (5 a.m.-7 a.m.)	Depressions above the kidneys
23	Midnight (II p.m.-I a.m.)	Right and left calves
24	Late evening (9 p.m.-II p.m.)	Palms
25	Midnight (II p.m.-I a.m.)	Tongue
26	Pre-dawn (3 a.m.-5 a.m.)	Neck
27	Daybreak (5 a.m.-7 a.m.)	Right and left shoulders
28	Sunrise (7 a.m.-9 a.m.)	Genitals
29	Early afternoon (I p.m.-3 p.m.)	Eyeballs
30	Sunrise (7 a.m.-9 a.m.)	Entire body

v) Position of the protective energy in relation to critical periods of the day

One of the most popular systems of astrology considers the twelve periods of the day (such as the period of dawn associated with the rabbit) more critically important than factors such as the year and month, the days of the lunar month, and the days of the week. Therefore, in this context, the position of the protective energy in relation to the twelve periods of the day should be given the most weight. The following table illustrates how to identify in which part of the body the protective energy of an individual resides in relation to the twelve periods of each day. It is important to avoid applying any kind of major external therapy to this locations at these times since it may damage the protective energy of an individual.

Correspondences Between the Protective Energy & the Twelve Periods

Period of the day	Location of Protective Energy
Daybreak (5 a.m.-7 a.m.)	Feet
Sunrise (7 a.m.-9 a.m.)	Neck, mouth
Mid-morning (9 a.m.-11 a.m.)	Occipital depression, lips
Midday (11 a.m.-1 p.m.)	Chest, eyes
Early afternoon (1 p.m.-3 p.m.)	Navel, uvula
Late afternoon (3 p.m.-5 p.m.)	Heart region
Sunset (5 p.m.-7 p.m.)	Spinal column
Early evening (7 p.m.-9 p.m.)	Both feet
Late evening (9 p.m.-11 p.m.)	Genitals
Midnight (11 p.m.-1 a.m.)	Stomach, genitals
After midnight (1 a.m.-3 a.m.)	Chest, stomach
Pre-dawn (3 a.m.-5 a.m.)	Intestines

II. VIṢṬI

Viṣṭi is one of the eleven actions[27] related to the course of the planets and stars of zodiacal astrology.[28] It is negative if strong external therapies and treatments coincide with the time during which the *viṣṭi* influence is present. The following table illustrates the days of the lunar month and general times of the day when the *viṣṭi* influence is present. It is important to avoid applying any kind of major external therapy at these times since it may damage the protective energy of an individual.

Days of the Lunar Month	Time of Presence
4, 11, 18, 25	Afternoon
8, 15, 22, 29	Morning

III. Nāga Kulika

The following table illustrates the earlier and latter parts of the twelve periods of the day — such as at daybreak on a particular day — when the *Nāga Kulika* influence is present. It is important to avoid applying any kind of major external therapy or treatment[29] at these times since it may damage the protective energy of an individual.

Periods When the Influence of the Nāga Kulika Is Present

Day of the Week	Period of Nāga Kulika
Sunday	Latter mid-morning (10 a.m.-11 a.m.) Late afternoon (3 p.m.-5 p.m.) Latter late evening (10 p.m.-11 p.m.) Pre-dawn (3 a.m.-5 a.m.)
Monday	Latter part of daybreak (6 a.m.-7 a.m.) Early afternoon (1 p.m.-3 p.m.) After midnight (1 a.m.-3 a.m.)
Tuesday	Midday (11 a.m.-1 p.m.) Early afternoon (1 p.m.-3 p.m.) Early evening (7 p.m.-9 p.m.) After midnight (1 a.m.-3 a.m.)
Wednesday	Sunrise (7 a.m.-9 a.m.) Midday (11 a.m.-1 p.m.) Midnight (11 p.m.-1 a.m.)
Thursday	Mid-morning to early midday (9 a.m.-12 p.m.) Late evening to midnight (9 p.m.-1 a.m.)
Friday	Latter sunrise to mid-morning (8 a.m.-11 a.m.) Latter early evening (8 p.m.-9 p.m.)
Saturday	Daybreak to sunrise (5 a.m.-9 a.m.) Early evening to late evening (7 p.m.-11 p.m.)

The Auspicious Mantra for Eliminating Negative Consequences

In cases where moxa or other therapies have to be performed at a time or place in discord with the position of the protective energy, all major texts of Tibetan medicine say that the following profound mantra will eliminate the related negative consequences:[30]

ༀ་ཚཀྵུ་དེ་བ་ཧྲི་མ་གི་སྭ་ཧཱ།

OM TSAKSHU DEVA HRI MA GI SVA HA

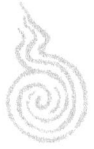

Appendix B

ABOUT THE AUTHOR

Chögyal Namkhai Norbu[1] was born in 1938 in Derge in eastern Tibet and was soon after recognized as a Buddhist reincarnate or *tulku* of high rank.[2] In fifty years as a member of the Tibetan diaspora, he has become a world figure as a master of Dzogchen, the Great Perfection, a body of ancient spiritual knowledge recognized as the supreme vehicle of Tibetan Buddhism.[3] He is also a renowned scholar of the culture of Tibet, with particular emphasis on its early history and on the systems of medicine and astrology originating from the Bön, pre-Buddhist, spiritual traditions that flourished in the kingdom of Shang Shung and from there spread throughout Tibet. This brief biography focuses, in the context of this manual, on the author's medical background, one aspect of his vast body of knowledge and expertise.

The education Chögyal Namkhai Norbu received in his early years in Tibet, taught by eminent masters of his time, encompassed the traditional array of subjects counted among the five sciences (Buddhist philosophy, medicine, logic, language and grammar, and arts and crafts). Already as a child, he received teachings on important Dzogchen texts from his maternal uncle Jamyang Khyentse Chökyi Wangchug[4] and his paternal uncle Togden Ugyen Tendzin.[5] The latter also gave him extensive oral instructions on the practice of Yantra Yoga.[6]

When Chögyal Namkhai Norbu entered Öntöd Sakya college at the age of nine, his teacher was Khenpo Khyenrab Chökyi Öser,[7] a renowned scholar of Buddhist philosophy and Tibetan medicine who was also the abbot of Öntöd.[8] One of his principal teachers was the famous Khenpo Shenga Rinpoche, an important figure in the nonsectarian (*rimé*) movement who revitalized scholarship in much of eastern Tibet.[9] Khyenrab Öser was a remarkable personage who, prevented by his parents from becoming a monk at the age of seven, ran away from home when he was thirteen to enroll in Öntöd monastery. Medicine and astrology were among the first subjects Khyenrab Öser studied, and, alongside Sutra, Tantra, and Dzogchen, remained throughout his life an important aspect of his erudition. A practicing physician and a leading authority on the *Four Medical Tantras*, he communicated this knowledge to Chögyal Namkhai Norbu.

Both learned and exceptionally kindhearted, Khyenrab Öser was a true bodhisattva, as he is called by the author. Colleges in Tibet did not generally provide food to students; at most there would be a simple kitchen for making tea. For anything beyond tea, students depended on family members or other benefactors. Mostly surviving on *tsampa*, Tibet's staple food, the young scholars mixed ground roasted barley with butter and hot tea to form a kind of porridge. Not realizing his ample supply was a finite quantity, the author would share his food with hungry fellow students and so found himself eventually without sustenance. Moreover, for lack of butter he was unable to make the butter lamps he needed for evening studies. Aware of his student's predicament, every evening Khyenrab Öser would give the author enough butter to make lamps for an hour or two of light. Having discovered that he would be given a bowl of barley soup in addition to the butter if he went to see his teacher around mealtime, the author made it a point to time his visits to Khyenrab Öser with that in mind. Day after day, his teacher unreservedly shared both butter and soup.

Khyenrab Öser's death was as remarkable as his life. In 1958, arrested by Chinese soldiers, he was being conducted to a public trial that would have certainly concluded in his execution. As his captors led him past a boulder known as Rock of the Noble Deer, he asked to rest for a moment. Granted his request, he sat on the rock, and, pronouncing HIK, performed the yogic transference of consciousness called phowa, dying instantly.

The second teacher to guide the author in the study of Tibetan medicine, again with an emphasis on the *Four Medical Tantras*, was Bo Kangkar Rinpoche Shedrub Chökyi Senge.[10] A brilliant scholar known both for his unsurpassed knowledge and noble character, he was a monk in the Kagyü tradition of Tibetan Buddhism and came from the culturally unique Kham-Minyag region of the eastern Tibetan plateau. He was educated in the nonsectarian style that was beginning to gain ground in the early twentieth century. Khenpo Shenga Rinpoche, the main master of Khyenrab Öser, was one of Kangkar Rinpoche's main teachers as well. Kangkar Rinpoche was tutor to H.H. the 16th Karmapa and had a very close student-teacher relationship with him. He was one of the first Tibetan lamas to teach students from other cultures, in particular China, and inspired some of the first teachers in the Tibetan tradition who taught in the West. He was also devoted to the dissemination of knowledge about Tibetan culture and history.

In the early 1950s, after Kangkar Rinpoche was held under house arrest in Dartsendo for many months, he was obliged to accept a position as a professor of Tibetan in his own monastery at Minyag Kangkar. The local government asked Chögyal Namkhai Norbu, then scarcely sixteen years old but already a graduate of Öntöd college, to assist him. Aware of the fact that Kangkar Rinpoche held a lineage of transmission of the *Four Medical Tantras* that came through the great master Jamgön Kongtrul,[11] Chögyal Namkhai Norbu requested that he be taught those texts again. While working at the school, he was able to see Kangkar Rinpoche every morning for lessons on medicine. During the same period, the author also received many teachings on Mahamudra and Dzogchen from that great lama.

By this time, although Chögyal Namkhai Norbu had twice studied the *Four Medical Tantras* thoroughly and gained general theoretical knowledge of Tibetan medicine, he still lacked practical experience. Then, at the age of eighteen, he met his teacher Nyala Rinpoche Rigdzin Changchub Dorje, an important Dzogchen master who was also a gifted doctor. During his life, Rigdzin Changchub Dorje received the revelation of special hidden treasure teachings on medicine, but practiced ordinary medicine as well and was an expert in that field.

Although Changchub Dorje was a Dzogchen master, outwardly he was a simple and modest person who lived as a country doctor. He led a community of Dzogchen practitioners at Khamdogar in the Dedrol area of Kham. His disciples also lived in an ordinary way, with few possessions, growing crops and tending animals, working on the land and practicing together.

Since he was well known in the area for his skills as a doctor, as many as a hundred people came to visit him daily for medical treatment or general advice. Only a few were aware that Rigdzin Changchub Dorje was a highly realized being and requested teachings from him or advice on subjects like meditation.

Having first dreamed about this extraordinary master, and then learned of his actual existence, Chögyal Namkhai Norbu traveled four days on horseback to his village to meet him. Introducing himself and telling the master about his background, he also mentioned that he had studied the *Four Medical Tantras* twice. Changchub Dorje's response was that now that he had learned all these subjects intellectually, it was time for him to apply them. To this end, the master had the author assist his medical students in performing therapies such as bloodletting and moxibustion for his many patients.

As part of his training, Chögyal Namkhai Norbu would go to the mountains, forests, and isolated villages to pick medicinal herbs. The master's advanced students knew how to recognize these herbs and taught him how to collect and detoxify them.

The author's description of his duties as his master's secretary aptly conveys a sense of Rigdzin Changchub Dorje's exceptional qualities: "Since Master Changchub Dorje hardly knew how to read and could not write, I offered myself as scribe whenever he had something to dictate. He asked me to transcribe the second volume of an important Dzogchen text he had received in a vision.[12] For days at a time, the master would dictate this text amid the constant stream of patients and other visitors. Time and again, the dictation was interrupted. I thought the result would be fragmented and lack continuity. Nevertheless, in the evening, when I read what I had written during the day, I was astounded by the perfection of the style and form of what he had dictated. Not a single word was missing, and it seemed as though it had been transmitted without any interruptions, which was all the more surprising considering that Master Changchub Dorje did not know how to write."[13]

In the late 1950s, Chögyal Namkhai Norbu made several pilgrimages to Central Tibet, India, Nepal, Sikkim, and Bhutan. During this period, Tibet was plunged into a steadily deepening condition of chaos in the aftermath of Chinese invasion. In 1959, while the author was in Sikkim, China's vehement response to the Tibetan population's uprising against its occupation made it impossible for him to return to his homeland. He stayed in Sikkim, writing and editing for the local government.

A brilliant young scholar, in 1960 he was invited to Rome, Italy, by Professor Giuseppe Tucci, an eminent figure in Italian Tibetological studies in the second third of the last century, as his collaborator at the ISMEO (Institute for Studies of the Middle and Extreme Orient). In 1962, at the age of twenty-three, Chögyal Namkhai Norbu became professor of Tibetan and Mongolian language and literature at the Institute of Oriental Studies at the University of Naples, a position that would last thirty years, until 1992.

In the mid-1970s, Chögyal Namkhai Norbu began teaching the Dzogchen point of view, meditation, and behavior, leading retreats and giving lectures on six continents, to an ever growing body of students. In 1981 he founded the International Dzogchen Community, a worldwide association composed of those interested in the knowledge and practice of this ancient spiritual path.

In 1988, Chögyal Namkhai Norbu established ASIA (Association for International Solidarity in Asia),[14] which implements projects of cooperation in Tibet as well as in other regions of the world. ASIA focuses its attention on the minority populations that are at greatest risk, such as the Tibetan nomads, working primarily in the sectors of education, health, and emergency disaster relief, providing aid to some of the most impoverished people on the planet. One of its most successful projects, Long Distance Sponsorship, serves some 1,500 individuals and provides access to modern education for children and youth in their native language, traditional Buddhist training for monks and nuns, training for Tibetan youth in traditional fine arts, performing arts, and literature, and dignified housing and services for displaced elderly Tibetans now living in India.

Among recent disaster relief efforts, ASIA has been providing basic necessities and education support to thousands of displaced victims in the wake of the 2010 earthquake disaster in Yushu Prefecture (traditionally the Kham region of

Tibet). ASIA, as a nonpolitical humanitarian organization, has worked continuously in Tibet for the past twenty-three years.

In 1991, in the presence of H.H. the Fourteenth Dalai Lama, Chögyal Namkhai Norbu inaugurated the International Shang Shung Institute of Tibetan Studies as a vehicle for the preservation of Tibetan culture in its manifold forms. The Institute's Ka-ter Translation Project was initiated for the translation and publication of the works of Chögyal Namkhai Norbu, the *terma* teachings of Rigdzin Changchub Dorje, and the Dzogchen tantras as well as the training of translators from Tibetan. Other endeavors of the Shang Shung Institute include the study of Tibetan traditional medicine, with an emphasis on practical training in the external therapies of moxibustion and kunye massage.[15] In 2005, the Shang Shung Institute's School of Tibetan Medicine[16] in Conway, Massachusetts, launched the world's first four-year Tibetan medicine program in English, adopting the curriculum of traditional schools of Tibetan medicine in Tibet and India. The program encompasses the *Four Medical Tantras* as well as Tibetan language, astrology, moxibustion, kunye massage therapy, ethics, and the history of traditional Tibetan medical practice.

Translated into all major languages, the author's numerous books, recordings, and films center on many aspects of the Dzogchen teaching as well as on the ancient history of Tibet and the medicine, astrology, and Yantra Yoga of that extraordinary culture. These materials are available through Shang Shung Institute, based at Merigar, Arcidosso, the seat of the Dzogchen Community in Italy.

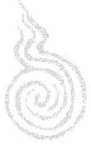

Notes

In the following notes, ChNN (Chögyal Namkhai Norbu) indicates information communicated orally by the author. Where relevant, Tibetan names and terms are given in Wylie transliteration to facilitate their identification.

ABOUT THIS BOOK

1   Rigdzin Changchub Dorje (*Byang chub rdo rje*, 1826-1961) is the root master of the author. Bo Kangkar Rinpoche Shedrub Chökyi Senge (*'Bo gangs dkar bshad sgrub chos kyi seng ge*, 1893-1957) was an exceptionally learned and famous master and the teacher of the 16th Karmapa. Khyenrab Öser (*mKhyen rab 'od zer*, 1889-1958) was a teacher, prolific author, and practicing doctor when the author was studying at Ontöd Sakya college in eastern Tibet. See Appendix B, About the Author.

TRANSLATOR'S INTRODUCTION

1   Shang Shung, an ancient kingdom in the region of Guge in western Tibet, is considered the source of Tibetan civilization. Shang Shung history is said to have had its origin more than 3,900 years ago, when the founder of the Everlasting Bön, Shenrab Miwoche (*gShen rab mi bo che*), made his appearance. In this context it is important to make a distinction between the Bön taught by Shenrab Miwoche (referred to as Everlasting Bön [*g.Yung drung bon*]) and the various Bönpo traditions that preceded Shenrab. Considering that Bön actually predated Shenrab Miwoche, there is basically no way to determine the origin of the first Bön lineages and hence the first Shang Shung generations from a historical perspective. See Appendix A, note 12, and Chögyal Namkhai Norbu, *The Light of Kailash*.

2   The word moxa is commonly believed to have originated from the Japanese term *mogusa* (艾), which is virtually identical to *moxa* in pronunciation since the *u* is not strongly enunciated. Chinese uses the same character as *mogusa*, but the single-syllable sound of the word (*ài*) is not related. It is possible that the Japanese term was adopted from the Tibetan *metsa*.

3   According to Tibetan medicine, the body is composed of three different energies or

humors (Wind, Bile, and Phlegm). Throughout this manual, the terms Wind, Bile, and Phlegm have been capitalized when referring to the three humors. Similarly, Blood has been capitalized when it represents a fourth humor in the ancient Bön system. See pp. xxiv to xxv, Basic Principles of Tibetan Medicine.

4   See note 3 above.

5   In this case, we are referring both to Bile energy (indicated by the capital B) and bile, the liquid secreted by the liver.

6   Tib. *tel* and *tshug*.

7   The herb traditionally used in Tibet is *spra ba* (pronounced *trawa*), generally translated as *Leontopodium franchetii*. Like edelweiss (*Leontopodium alpinum*), its leaves are covered in fine, whitish hairs. Its flowers are pale yellow. Although both the genus Artemisia and Leontopodium are in the Asteraceae family, *spra ba* is not identical to the *A. verlotiorum* traditionally used in Chinese and Japanese moxibustion, and it is not clear whether its medicinal properties are the same. See Thinley Gyatso, Chris Hakim, *Essentials of Tibetan Traditional Medicine*, North Atlantic Books, Berkeley, 2010.

8   For instance, artemisia can be mixed with nutmeg for Wind disorders, ginger for Phlegm, or pomegranate seed powder for digestive disorders.

9   See About This Book, note 1, and Part One, notes 60 and 61.

10   Tib. *yan lag*.

11   Tib. *'dus so*.

12   Tib. *chu ser*. See Part One, note 20, Part Two, note 157.

13   See Part Two, note 3, for more information on the Tibetan method of counting vertebrae.

14   It goes without saying that physical proportions vary from person to person. Accordingly, in some cases the location of the points shown in the drawings in this book may not always represent the actual position of a point on the body of an individual. It is therefore imperative to measure and locate each point as described in the individual listings in this manual. See Part One, p. 8.

15   See Part Two, notes 4 and 77.

16   See Part One, p. 9.

17   Tib. *bla*. See Appendix A, note 2.

18   Tib. *grib* and *gdon*, respectively. See Part One, note 27, and Part Two, notes 46, 47, 54, and 148.

19   The Yantra Yoga system of Vairochana is one of the oldest systems of Tibetan yoga. The author has written an extensive commentary on the root teachings by Vairochana from the eighth century, "Union of the Sun and Moon" (*Nyi zla kha sbyor*), based on the personal training and knowledge of Yantra Yoga he received from his uncle Togden Ugyen Tendzin and various other teachers in Tibet. Chögyal Namkhai Norbu began teaching Yantra Yoga in Italy in the early 1970s. See Chögyal Namkhai Norbu, *Yantra*

Yoga, and Chögyal Namkhai Norbu, *Rainbow Body* (a biography of Togden Ugyen Tendzin).

20 In effect, Tibetan astrology is based on the unification of a number of different systems, chiefly elemental astrology (*'byung rtsis*), also referred to as black astrology (*nag rtsis*), and zodiacal astrology (*skar rtsis*), also called white astrology (*dkar rtsis*). The latter, of Indian origin, was introduced in Tibet in 1027 and is far closer to Western sidereal and planetary astrology. See Chögyal Namkhai Norbu, *The Light of Kailash*.

PART ONE

1 *bDud rtsi snying po gsang ba man ngag gi rgyud*, traditionally referred to as the *rGyud chung*, is found in *Cha lag bco brgyad*. It is the earlier recension of what we now know as the *rGyud bzhi*. See notes 41 and 56 below.

2 Tib. *dpyad* or *dpyad lnga*.

3 Bloodletting (*gtar kha*), moxibustion (*me btsa'*), medical baths (*lums*), stone and compress therapy (*dugs*), and massage (*byugs pa* or *bku mnye*). In bloodletting, which is performed for three days, medicine is first administered to the patient to separate the pure from impure blood, and incisions are then made in specific veins. Medical baths are a form of heat therapy that involves taking baths in water in which medicinal substances have been dissolved. In stone therapy, hot or cold stones are applied to different parts of the body, depending on the nature of the illness. There are seventy-five or seventy-six different kinds of stones. In a similar therapy, hot compresses are applied using a piece of cotton pad that has been heated. In massage, creams and ointments are first applied to the skin and the therapist then kneads the body using various techniques. For a presentation of Tibetan massage techniques, see Chögyal Namkhai Norbu, *The Practice of Tibetan Kunye Massage*.

4 The herb traditionally used in Tibet was *spra ba*. See Translator's Introduction, note 7.

5 The auspicious days for collecting herbs are days when favorable astrological combinations occur. See Appendix A, notes 1 and 7.

6 The beginning, middle, and end of autumn, roughly corresponding to September, October, and November. After picking, the herbs are washed lightly in a stream or water source located in the place where they were found.

7 Bruising the herb serves the purpose of letting its sap seep out a little to mix it with the outer part of the plant.

8 Herbs are generally dried in the shade or in the sun according to the nature of the herb. Most herbs of a hot nature, used as a remedy for cold disorders, should be dried in the sun, while most herbs of a cold nature, used as a remedy for hot disorders, should be dried in the shade. Some herbs are also dried in the wind. Notwithstanding the fact that moxibustion is used to treat cold disorders, Tibetan practice calls for drying *spra ba* in the shade. See also Translator's Introduction, note 7.

9   This is to make the herb softer and easier to press into cones or balls.

10   Tib. *thang shing,* a specific species of pine.

11   After rolling the moxa in thin rice paper or cigarette paper, it is cut in half to create two cones. See images on p. 4 and Translator's Introduction, p. xiii.

12   See "Methods of Applying Moxibustion" below.

13   Salt or a slice of ginger or garlic and other medicinal ingredients can also be used as a support. In this case, the cone is placed on top of the support, which forms a barrier between the skin and the cone. See Translator's Introduction, p. xv, and note 49 below.

14   Loss of metabolic heat (*me drod nyams pa*) can be indicated, for example, by poor or difficult digestion.

15   In Tibetan medicine, *skya bab,* translated here as first-stage edema, denotes a Phlegm-related disorder whose primary causes are the same as those that cause disorders of Phlegm in general. Its secondary causes are failure to digest nutritive essence and an accumulation of undigested nutritive essence in the liver leading to an increase of impure blood and lymph. General symptoms include pallor and swellings.

16   Third-stage edema (*dmu chu*) is characterized by the abnormal accumulation of fluids in cells, tissues, or cavities of the body, resulting in swellings. It is caused by a lack of assimilation of foods, excessive treatments of a cold nature, loss of digestive heat, the patient's past actions, or provocations from *nāgas,* and so forth. Its general symptoms include weakness; a sensation of abdominal fullness; panting; palpitations; pale tongue, gums, and lips; abdominal heaviness during movement; and swelling in eight areas of the body: top of the foot, shin, third lumbar vertebra, abdomen, chest, face, mouth, and eyelids.

17   In Tibetan medicine, *skran,* the term for tumor, includes many types of new tissue growth that can be varied in nature: bilious; epigastric; of the blood; of the blood vessels; of the uterus and ovaries; of fluid; of calculi; of microorganisms; of ingested matter; and so on. The condition arises from the following primary causes: poor digestion; imbalances of Phlegm, Bile, Wind, or Blood; microorganisms; lymphatic disorders; or ingestion of hair. Trauma, wounds from weapons, childbirth, residing in cold places, past actions, and energetic disturbances are secondary causes.

18   Tib. *'bras.* Cysts are an abnormal structure or pocket filled with fluids or disused matter, including abscesses. According to Tibetan medicine, they can be caused by trauma, imbalance of the three humors, poor assimilation of foods, or residual blood. They can manifest on the surface of the body or internally.

19   Tib. *grang mkhris.* Disorders of this type are accompanied by symptoms such as poor digestion and a whitish color of the feces.

20   Lymphatic disorders (*chu ser kyi nad*) are illnesses related to lymph or serum. Lymph (*chu ser*) refers to the sticky fluid primarily located below the skin and in the joints. After the nutriment of food is transformed into blood, its waste product accumulates in the gallbladder, further separating into lymph and bile. The pure part of the bile is

digestive bile, the impure part is excreted in the urine. See *Dictionary of Healing Arts* (*gSo ba rig pa'i mdzod g.yu thog dgongs rgyan*), pp. 167-168, Translator's Introduction p. xix, and Part Two, notes 157 and 160.

21   In Tibetan medicine, poor digestion (*ma zhu ba*) is considered the cause of internal illnesses. It is primarily due to an increase of cold Phlegm in the body. Its secondary causes include a constitution that predisposes one to such a disorder, a diet to which one is not accustomed, or foods that are incompatible or difficult to digest. Poor digestion can be related to various conditions and presents the following general symptoms: constipation, irregular evacuation of bowels, abdominal distension, constipation followed by diarrhea, heaviness, loss of appetite, malaise after meals, belching, headaches, and apathy.

22   Epigastric disorders (*lhen nad*) are characterized by the abnormal formation of gastric mucus in the stomach process caused by the loss of digestive heat and poor digestion. These disorders are accompanied by pain and a sense of obstruction in the upper part of the stomach, loss of appetite, malaise after meals, and difficulty in digestion.

23   Chronic gastritis (*lcags dreg*) is a Phlegm-related illness defined as the adherence of gastric mucus to the wall of the stomach and consequent obstruction of the secretion of gastric juices. It is caused by loss of digestive heat and poor digestion. The obstruction of the secretion of gastric juices diminishes the heat of the digestive Bile, causing the manifestation of the following symptoms: belching, a sensation of fullness, diffused pain in the stomach, loss of appetite, loss of weight, laziness, and vomiting of mucus or undigested food. Iron rust, the literal translation of the name of this illness, refers to a distinctive rust-like stain in the abdominal region.

24   Empty fever (*stong tshad*) refers to a pathological increase of bodily temperature associated with Wind. While its primary cause is Wind, the secondary causes for this type of fever can be of different kinds. These can be naturally occurring or related to the circumstances or to the particular seat of an illness: for example, an illness of a hot nature; an illness in which Wind is predominant; a cold and windy place; the humid part of summer or autumn; old age; a Wind constitution; fever associated with malaise in the lumbar region; treatment with medicines of an excessively cold nature; or a fever affecting the vital channels.

25   According to Tibetan medicine, insanity (*smyo byed*) is a disorder caused by a weakness of spirit, sorrow, dissatisfaction, and excessive mental activity, but also by diet and behavior incompatible with one's constitution and by sudden provocations of energy. Seven types are explained in Tibetan medicine: due to Wind, Bile, and Phlegm separately; due to these three together; due to suffering; due to intoxication or poisoning; or due to provocations. Each type is distinguished by different symptoms.

26   The Tibetan term for epilepsy (*brjed byed*) literally refers to an illness causing forgetfulness. Its causes are the same as those leading to insanity. General symptoms include

palpitations, dizziness, profuse sweating, abdominal distension, weakness, stiffness of the limbs, difficulty in bending the limbs, abundant salivation and mucus, fainting at the manifestation of the illness, clenching of the teeth, shaking of the legs, vomiting of bubbly liquid, dimmed perception, obscured eyesight, and epileptic seizures.

27   Illnesses caused by provocations (*gdon nad*) are of different natures. They can be caused by factors such as the disturbance of external elements or by spirits that can negatively influence one's energy. A similarly arcane source of disease is referred to as contamination (*grib*). See Translator's Introduction, pp. xxii to xxiii, and Part Two, notes 46, 47, 54, and 148.

28   Tib. *rtsa nad kyi rigs*. According to Tibetan medicine, neurological disorders are caused by the malfunction of the Wind humor that moves in opposite pathways and invades the nerves or blood vessels. This condition can occur because of trauma caused by strenuous activities; contagious diseases; intoxication and poisoning; fever; injury from weapons; or due to being beaten. Neurological disorders are distinguished by bodily location and the area with which they are associated.

29   According to Western medicine, gout is a hereditary form of arthritis resulting from a disturbance of uric acid in the metabolism, characterized by an excess of uric acid in the blood and deposits of uric acid salts, usually in the joints of the feet and hands, especially in the big toe. According to Tibetan medicine, gout (*dreg*) is caused by food and behavior that upset the blood, excessive exposure to heat, sleeping during the daytime, remaining inactive after ingesting nutrient-rich foods, and doing activities that require great physical effort.

30   Arthritis and rheumatoid arthritis (*gram bu*) are, according to Tibetan medicine, illnesses of a cold nature caused by dwelling in cold and damp places and excessive consumption of fatty foods. As a result, lymph deposits itself in tissues, bones, blood vessels, tendons, and ligaments, manifesting symptoms such as pain in the muscles and joints characterized by inflammation, and stiffness, aching pain (especially at night), and difficulty in walking and stretching the legs and limbs. It is classified into arthritis of the tissue; of the bones and of the blood vessels; of the tendons and ligaments; and of a cold and hot nature. An effective remedy for rheumatoid arthritis is to eat raw, still warm pork liver.

31   Although moxibustion is not indicated in the presence of a strong fever, it can be used in the case of persistent, low-grade fevers.

32   Wounds (*rma*) caused by accidents, and the like.

33   Anthrax (*lhog pa*) is an infectious disease related to microorganisms naturally present in the blood. It occurs when these microorganisms are altered by secondary causes such as an environment where an epidemic is taking place, infected animals, the season, diet, behavior, and provocations of energy. Depending on the nature of the pustules it presents, the disease is classified into eleven different types.

34   Warts (*'dzer pa*) are a skin disease that present hard growths of various kinds, such as verruca. Celidonia is said to be a good remedy for this problem.

35   Fever related to Bile (*mkhris tshad*) is caused by an imbalance of Bile.

36   Tib. *khrag nad*. See Translator's Introduction, p. xii.

37   The *Blue Beryl* (*Vaidurya sngon po*) of Desi Sangye Gyatso (*sDe srid sangs rgyas rgya mtsho;* 1653–1705), a detailed commentary on the *Four Medical Tantras*, explains that there are three channels in relation to the urinary bladder channels: "The urinary channel or urethra (*chu rtsa*), the life vessel (*srog rtsa*), and the procreation vessel (*srid rtsa*). These are located next to the sexual organs in men and women. In the center is the urine channel, so called because urine flows in it. On the right is the life vessel, so called because in it flows Wind energy, and on the left is the vessel of procreation, so called because in it flows the semen in men and the blood element in woman." *gSo ba rig pa'i tshig mdzod g.yu thog dgons rgyan*, pp. 641-642.

38   Tib. *mig rtsa*.

39   In the original Tibetan text, the discussion of astrological factors was included in Part One. The specifications referred to here apply in particular to the cauterization and burning methods of moxa, but if these prescriptions are followed in milder moxa applications, the treatment can be more effective.

40   See "Methods of Applying Moxa" below for the definition of these methods of treatment.

41   The *Last Tantra* is the last of the *Four Medical Tantras* (*rGyud bzhi*). The *rGyud bzhi* is a four-volume treatise consisting of the *Root Tantra* (*rTsa ba'i rgyud*), *Explanatory Tantra* (*bShad pa'i rgyud*), *Secret Oral Instruction Tantra* (*Man ngag gi rgyud*), and *Last Tantra* (*Phyi ma'i rgyud*). To date, only the first two volumes have been published in English (as *The Quintessence Tantras of Tibetan Medicine*, trans. Dr. Barry Clark, Snow Lion Publications, Ithaca, NY, 2005). A bilingual English-Tibetan edition of the first two volumes was published in 2009 by Men-Tsee-Khang Institute under the title *Basic Tantra and the Explanatory Tantra from the Secret Quintessential Instructions on the Eight Branches of the Ambrosia Essence Tantra*. Men-Tsee-Khang intends to publish a translation of the remaining two volumes in the future. An earlier version, *The Ambrosia Heart Tantra: A Classic Treatise on Tibetan Medicine*, annotated by Dr. Yeshi Dhonden and translated by B. Allan Wallace, may now be out of print (Library of Tibetan Works & Archives, 1976 and 1995). See also note 56 below.

42   See Translator's Introduction, note I, and p. 11.

43   Scalpel (*thur ma*): a general term for a class of traditional Tibetan surgical instruments, as those used in bloodletting or in the case of pericardial effusion; sometimes an acupuncture needle.

44   Cauterizing (*btso ba*), burning (*sreg pa*), heating (*bsro ba*), and threatening (*sdig pa*).

45   The moxibustion method of cauterization is not easy to apply. It should only be used on patients who are critically ill. The medical texts say that in these cases the moxa

cone should be larger than usual. Moreover, while it is burning, the doctor blows on the cone until it has burned away completely. At the end, with the sound *tsak*, a small piece of seared skin cracks away. This method should be applied only by a practitioner who has extensive knowledge and experience of moxibustion. The cauterization method is used five, seven, or even twelve times in a single session. Among the five hundred points listed in this manual, cauterization is only applied to the points where such treatment is expressly specified, that is, the points on the central and lateral back. It may also be applied with extreme care on certain localized points. See Translator's Introduction, p. xvi.

46   Pale Phlegm (*bad kan skya bo*) refers to Phlegm-related illnesses of an exclusively cold nature. See Part Two, note 15.

47   Depressive syndrome (*snying rlung*), literally heart-wind disease, an illness caused by an imbalance of the Wind that affects the earth element. The symptoms include trembling, a sensation as if the chest were filled with air, yawning, mental confusion and instability, senseless speech, dizziness, and insomnia. See Part Two, notes 6, 23, and 86.

48   The same precautions referred to in connection with cauterization apply to burning (see Translation's Introduction, pp. xii, xiv, and xxi, note 45 above, and pp. 5, 6, and 8. However, the moxibustion method of burning does not require the skin to be burned directly as is done in the cauterizing method. See note 49 below.

49   When using the burning method, the moxa cone can be placed on a support consisting of a layer of salt, a slice of ginger, a slice of garlic, or other appropriate medicinal substance. Even though the skin is not burned directly, the heat generated is still very high. (ChNN) Supports can also be used for the heating or threatening methods of application. See Translator's Introduction, p. xv, and note 13 above for a discussion of indirect moxa using supports.

50   A variety of pathologies are included in this disorder, for instance urine and water retention and blood obstructing blood vessels. (ChNN)

51   For instance, using moxa sticks or supports. See note 49 above.

52   Firmly placing the thumb right on the spot where the moxibustion was applied, one does a little massage without rubbing the skin. This is also beneficial following the application of the last two methods of moxibustion. (ChNN) Additionally, it is helpful to put a little salted butter or other appropriate cream on the points that have been treated.

53   If you feel very thirsty after a couple of hours you can drink hot tea, for example, but no cold drinks. (ChNN)

54   For the therapies that use burning with a metal instrument called *tel* or *tsug* in Tibetan medicine, and for the cauterization type of moxibustion, these guidelines must be followed for seven days; otherwise the efficacy of the moxa will be undermined. (ChNN)

See Translator's Introduction, p. xxi.

55 In departure from standard editorial practice, titles of unpublished translations in English have been italicized.

56 Some scholars assert that the *rGyud bzhi* was composed in India and then translated into Tibetan, though others disagree with this theory. In fact, in the *Four Medical Tantras*, we find various names of medicinal herbs and other terms, unrelated to the Indian system, in the ancient language of Shang Shung. This suggests that there was an indigenous medical literature in Tibet. If such literature did not exist, we could not explain the presence of many Shang Shung words in the *Four Medical Tantras*. Moreover, a number of ancient medical books are mentioned in early Bön writings. Although the books themselves have not been found, this confirms that medical knowledge had already been discovered at that point. Tibetan history tells us that the ancient Tibetan kings invited many doctors from various countries, and as a result of their meetings committed their knowledge to writing. This would explain why we find elements from many different traditions in Tibetan medicine. At a later time, the famous Tibetan doctor Yutog Yönten Gönpo gathered medical knowledge from different sources and may have compiled the *Four Medical Tantras*. Whatever the case may be, the *Four Medical Tantras* is considered the most important treatise of Tibetan medicine. It formed the basis for the description of the majority of the moxibustion points given here. (ChNN) Two outstanding doctors by the name Yutog Yönten Gönpo (*g.Yu thog yon tan mgon po*) appeared in Tibet. The one referred to here is Yutog Yönten Gönpo the Elder, who lived in the eighth century (708-833). Yutog Yönten Gönpo the Younger (1126-1202) is said to have revised and expanded the *Four Medical Tantras* on the basis of their existing transmission lineages. See also note 41 above.

57 The authorship of *Zla ba'i rgyal po* is rather complicated. It is generally attributed to Nāgārjuna under the Sanskrit title *Somarājabhaisajyasādhanā*. See note 58 below.

58 The version of *The Moon King* translated directly from Sanskrit into Tibetan by the great translator and spiritual master Vairochana and the version translated into Tibetan from the Chinese should be the same, but on close examination the two texts have slight differences in the verses and other areas. For example, in *The Moon King* translated by Vairochana we do not find some moxibustion points that are mentioned in the version translated from the Chinese. (ChNN)

59 Tun-Huang, sometimes spelled Dunhuang, is a city in central Asia, now in the Gansu province of China. In ancient times, Tun-Huang was a major point of communication between ancient China and Central Asia with a large and important library. For many centuries, the town, together with the library, was submerged by the sands of the desert. Later, the site was rediscovered along with many important documents and books in Chinese, Tibetan, and other Asian languages. The collection included texts on ancient history as well as on medicine and moxibustion. The two Tun-Huang

manuscripts on moxibustion referred to here (*Pelliot tibétain 127* and *Pelliot tibétain 1044*) are very ancient, as indicated by their pronounced divergence in style from modern Tibetan. In addition to explaining many of the moxibustion points that are in the *Four Medical Tantras*, they also mention several others.

60 Dilmar or De'u Mar Geshe Tenzin Phuntshog (*Dil dmar dge bshes bstan 'dzin phun tshogs*) lived in the seventeenth century (1672-?). A scholar extremely learned in all fields of knowledge, he was referred to as a pandit (*De'u dmar pan chen*). He was the author of many works on different subjects, especially medicine and pharmacology. Dilmar was also a spiritual master knowledgeable in both the Mahamudra and Dzogchen systems and the founder of the Dagpo Kagyü monastery of *De'u dmar zab rgyas chos gling*, in eastern Tibet. He had many students, among them the outstanding Situ Dharmakara. Rigdzin Changchub Dorje, the author's master, considered Dilmar a very important doctor and had different visions of him in which he received instructions. Dilmar's book on moxibustion, *The White Crystal Mirror: A Large Instruction on Moxibustion* (*Me btsa'i gdams pa rgyas spros shel dkar me long*) is one of the richest texts on this practice found in Tibet, and it contains many points that are not in the *Four Medical Tantras*. (ChNN)

61 The rediscovered treasure teachings on medicine such as *The Continuous Rainfall of Nectar That Preserves the Life of Beings* (*'Gro ba'i srog 'dzin bdud rtsi'i char rgyun*) are intended for curing illnesses of different epochs. For example, nowadays we have modern illnesses that did not exist in the past. Realized beings, such as Padmasambhava, who had knowledge of future events and methods of healing diseases with medicines and mantras, formulated and concealed teachings to be rediscovered at later times when these illnesses manifested. This is why medical teachings found in these rediscovered treasures can be very important. In Changchub Dorje's rediscovered treasure texts in particular, we find many points of moxibustion that are not mentioned in other manuals on the subject. (ChNN)

62 Khyungtrul Jigme Namkhai Dorje Yungdrung Gyaltsan (*Khyung sprul 'jigs med nam mkha'i rdo rje g.yung drung rgyal mtshan*, 1897-1955) was a spiritual master originally from the Kailash region and also very learned in medicine and astrology. The treatise referred to here mostly follows the explanations given in *The Last Tantra*, but we also find in it interesting variations possibly linked with ancient Bön medicine. (ChNN)

PART TWO

1 The Tibetan word *yan lag*, or limb, also includes the head.

2 The points along the spine generally consist of a central point and two lateral points, of which the central is the most important. See also Translation's Introduction, p. xx and note 4 below.

3 This, the first *an stong* in the *Byang* tradition of Tibetan medicine, corresponds to the seventh cervical vertebra in the Western medical system. The first six cervical vertebrae

are not called *an stong* in the Tibetan medical system. The lumbar and sacral vertebrae (*sked tshigs* and *tshang rus*) correspond with the Western system. In the following, the numbering of the "vertebrae" starts with the seventh cervical (Wind Point) as number one.

4 Moxa is performed directly on the spinous process of the vertebrae, not in the space between vertebrae. Application of moxa in the space between vertebrae could bring negative neurological consequences. If using Japanese-style moxa cones, it is possible to apply heat on all three points simultaneously. With Chinese moxa sticks, first apply heat to the central point, then to the one on the patient's right, and finally to the one to the left. (ChNN) See Translator's Introduction, p. xx, and note 77 below.

5 Bile (*mkhris pa*), Phlegm (*bad kan*), and Wind (*rlung*) constitute the triad of humors spoken of in Tibetan medicine as well as in Ayurveda. The principle of the three humors was probably already present in ancient Bön medicine. In fact, according to some sources, ancient Bön medicine made a distinction between four, not three, humors; the fourth was Blood (*khrag*). (ChNN) See also Translator's Introduction, pp. xxiii to xxv.

6 Here the insanity is caused by a depressive syndrome or *srog rlung nad* (life-sustaining Wind disorder; see Part One, note 47, and note 86 below). The life-sustaining Wind is one of the five Winds that govern the various functions of body and mind. The condition of *srog rlung nad* occurs when the life-sustaining Wind takes a wrong course and harms the functions of the white life channel (*srog rtsa*) or coronaries. Coronaries here translates the Tibetan *srog rtsa* (life channel). *Srog rtsa* stands for the channels that support the life force and are the root of all channels. There are two types: black (*srog rtsa nag po*) and white (*srog rtsa dkar po*). The black life channel refers to the coronaries that carry Blood and Wind combined. Implicitly, the black life channel could also indicate the vena cava. The white life channel is the spinal cord in which the life-sustaining Wind abides. It connects the brain to the coccyx. See *gSo ba rig pa'i tshig mdzod g.yu thog dgongs rgyan* (*Dictionary of Healing Arts*), pp. 645-46 and 647-48, where the term is rendered as coronaries. This seems to be the intended meaning in this context. The yogic practice related to channels and energy winds (*rtsa rlung*) and *kumbhaka* (*bum pa can*), for example, can cause this illness if applied without qualified guidance. More commonly this illness occurs in ordinary people.

7 A pale tongue is a sign of an imbalance of Wind or Phlegm. (ChNN)

8 Chronic fever (*tshad pa rnying pa*) can refer to persistent, low-grade fever or to a hidden fever condition that can reemerge at a later time.

9 The kind of back pain referred to here is caused by a disturbance of Wind or by high blood pressure caused by Wind. (ChNN)

10 Obstruction of the esophagus caused by Phlegm (*bad kan pho thog*) is defined as a shrinking of the esophagus due to an abnormal increase of phlegm in the stomach, chest, and lungs. This illness starts with the sensation of an obstruction in the

esophagus; eventually the swallowing of food becomes difficult. It can easily become aggravated and turn into either a cancer of the stomach or cancer of the esophagus. The symptoms of this illness include loss of appetite, breathing problems, loss of weight, loss of physical energy, and reduction in the size of the stomach. Nine different forms of this illness are discussed in Tibetan medicine. The best way to treat this problem is to apply moxa at its outset. See also notes 76 and 80 below.

11   The name of these points, Cold Bile (*grang mkhris*), refers to a Bile condition of a cold nature.

12   See Part One, note 19.

13   Goiter (*lba ba*) is distinguished in terms of its main cause and the form in which it presents itself. In Tibetan medicine, it is classified into eight types. The primary causes of goiter include diet, behavior, and an incorrect, excessive, or weak treatment of an illness. Its secondary causes are the malfunction of the blood vessels in the neck. One method of treating goiter is to insert heated needles in various points of the goiter and then extract them quickly. The process is repeated two or three times a week.

14   Wind of a cold nature (*grang rlung*) refers to a cold condition caused by Wind accompanied by symptoms such as a cold sensation in the abdominal region and waist, difficult digestion, and agitation when exposed to cold.

15   Pale Phlegm (*bad kan skya bo*) indicates an illness of Phlegm of a cold nature. Brown Phlegm (*bad kan smug po*) indicates Phlegm illnesses connected to an imbalance of all three humors that alters the normal condition of the blood, which at that point becomes the cause of the illness. It can affect the stomach, liver, intestines, and colon, but also the internal and surface parts of the body. Its symptoms include alternating pain in the stomach and intestines, pain radiating from the chest to the back, a foul smell in the mouth, heartburn, retching, headaches with pain around the eyes, excruciating pain when the body has cooled down after perspiring, dry and dark feces, malaise on an empty and full stomach, malaise when exposed to cold, unmotivated malaise, sudden improvement of one's condition, and manifestation of the illness in autumn and spring. Untreated over a long time, this condition can turn into cancer. Many forms of this illness are explained in detail in Tibetan medicine.

16   See note 13 above.

17   Contagious diseases (*rims nad*) such as the flu.

18   Tib. *glo ma*, lit. maternal lobes of the lungs.

19   Tib. *glo'i bu*, lit. filial lobes of the lungs. In some moxa manuals these points are called General Lung Points (*glo ba'i spyi gsang*).

20   A combined Phlegm and Wind (*bad rlung*) disorder causes dizziness and an unsteady gait.

21   Such as a severe flu.

22   See note 6 above.

23   Emotional instability (*shes pa 'phyo ba* or *snying 'phyo ba* or *sems 'phyo ba*) is also considered an

illness in which the person does not remain in a normal state but becomes confused and troubled. Such an illness manifests symptoms such as forgetfulness, moodiness, and un-motivated displeasure. People affected by this type of disturbance sometimes speak non-sense or do not reply when they are addressed. They become apprehensive upon hearing unpleasant words, have shortness of breath, sleep little, have a sensation that their heart is empty and that their upper back is full; in particular they feel pain at the point in be-tween the breasts and at the sixth and seventh vertebrae. If this problem persists, the per-son may feel pain throughout the body and fall unconscious. If untreated, over time it can result in depressive symptoms (*snying rlung*) and insanity.

24 See note 6 above.

25 People affected by this problem normally feel pain on an empty stomach or when they are hungry. They therefore have to eat frequently. (ChNN)

26 Weak liver illness (*mchin rgud kyi nad*) is essentially a Phlegm imbalance that affects the liver. Its symptoms include pain in the liver after meals, physical weakness, vomiting of hot liquids, and blocked yawning.

27 Sometimes spleen disorders can cause skin rashes. Such cases can also be treated with moxa on these points. (ChNN)

28 If the face becomes thinner while the flesh on the other parts of the body remains the same, it can be a sign of spleen disorder.

29 Tib. *lhen nad*. These disorders are caused by a deterioration of the digestive heat, for instance due to an increase of stomach mucus as a consequence of poor digestion.

30 See Part One, note 23.

31 See note 15 above.

32 Tib. *bsam se'u*: A general term for male and female reproductive organs.

33 Colic (*glang thabs*) can be caused by indigestion, eating unfamiliar foods or foods that do not agree with one's constitution (resulting in a kind of intoxication), or an imbal-ance of the stomach bacteria from exposure to cold after perspiring.

34 A blockage of the urine flow where urine is expelled in drops and with difficulty.

35 It is imperative not to apply moxa laterally to the central point because it could dam-age the function of the kidneys or the procreation channels (*srid rtsa*); cf. *Cha byad dpyad*.

36 Tib. *mo sman gyi ngan khrag rgyu ba*. This can refer to a variety of menstrual problems, such as heavy or frequent menstruation or trapped menstrual blood.

37 In this disorder, the mucus can present itself in various colors in the diarrhea.

38 The Tibetan term *chu so* can either refer to the tip of the urethra or the bladder. See *gSo ba rig pa'i tshig mdzod g.yu thog dgongs rgyan*, p. 168.

39 Downward-clearing Wind (*thur sel rlung*): One of the five principal Winds spoken of in Tibetan medicine and in the tantras. It controls the functions of the sexual organs and the lower parts of the body.

40 Tib. *gzhug chung ngam rta mig gi mjug*.

41   Includes sinusitis.

42   This illness can be caused by stress, tension, and worry. The typical symptoms are constriction and pain at the shoulder blades.

43   Tib. *rtsa grib*. The term refers to neurological disorders such as stroke and paralysis as well as less dramatic complaints such as loss of sensation, in particular as a result of planetary influences. See also Part One, note 27, and note 54 below.

44   As in the case of meningitis.

45   *Kalo* (*ka lo*): possibly a specific name for a bone in the head.

46   Provocations (*gdon*), external disturbances, environmental factors, or various types of malevolent beings that cause health problems. There are many types of illnesses linked to provocations; cancer, for example, is related to the influence of the class of beings called *btsan*. In this case, in addition to the standard medical treatment it is advisable for the patient to do the visualization and recitation of the mantras of Red Garuda or Hayagriva, deities that are related to the *btsan* class of beings. (ChNN) See also Translator's Introduction, pp. xxii to xxiii, Part One, note 27, and notes 47, 54, and 148 below.

47   Provocations from above (*steng gdon*) is a broad category of disturbances that includes conditions called shooting star disturbance (*skar mda'*), star provocation (*skar gdon*), and provocations related to astrological influences of the days of the week. It occurs, for example, to those who travel and sleep in open places and feel afraid while doing so. Because they are very similar to the symptoms of other diseases, such as stroke, epilepsy, and certain diseases related to contamination, the specific symptoms can only be identified by studying the individual's astrological chart. See also note 46 above.

48   Dilmar explains that because the Sanskrit term *yama* is homophonic with the word for a sinus disease in Shang Shung language, the class of beings called *yama* are sometimes considered to be responsible for this disease. In effect, however, these conditions are caused by specific microorganisms, also called *yama*, that can be of two types: white, characterized by a combination of Wind and Phlegm disorders, and black, characterized by a combination of Blood and Bile. See also note 46 above.

49   Gate of the Sky (*gnam sgo*): in this case sky also signifies above or upper.

50   Each five-point cluster (*lnga tshoms*) consists of the point itself and the four points one finger from the central point in the four intermediate directions.

51   Tib. *bad kan pho thog rigs dgu'i nad*. Even though the illness is initially concentrated in the esophagus, these obstructions present a great risk of spreading quickly if not treated with moxa.

52   Dilmar's *White Crystal* manual of moxibustion includes the central points under the name Ratna Points, but not the outer points in Changchub Dorje's system.

53   This is typically a needle-like pain radiating from the chest to the back. Among other things, this kind of pain can be caused by panic attacks and can be the starting point

of a heart attack.

54   Tib. *grib sgo'i gsang*. The term *grib* is generally translated as contamination here and includes visible and invisible environmental influences. In Tibetan culture, funerals (in particular of victims of certain diseases or violent deaths), childbirth, persons of a certain social status, discord, and other factors are considered potential sources of contamination, pollution, or defilement, and as such are believed to adversely affect the health of people exposed to them. See also Part One, note 27.

55   See Part One, note 27.

56   Called Black Tip in Dilmar's *White Crystal*.

57   Tib. *phrag mig*, lit. eye of the shoulder. Eye sometimes refers to a socket, but here it means central point, that is, the area where the principal function is located, which is also a sensitive area where finger pressure produces pain.

58   On the four points (*bzhi khrom*) means that in this case moxa is not applied on the central point but only on the four outer points of each cluster.

59   The five types of Wind (*rlung lnga*) are life-sustaining Wind (*srog 'dzin*); ascending Wind (*rgyen rgyu*); pervading Wind (*khyab byed*); fire-accompanying Wind (*me mnyam*); and downward-clearing Wind (*thur sel*). Each of these types of Wind performs specific functions within the body-mind complex. The life-sustaining Wind dwells mainly in the head, but circulates through the throat, chest, and nerves. It presides over swallowing, breathing, spitting, sneezing, and belching. It clarifies the eyes and other senses and sustains the cerebral functions. The ascending Wind dwells mainly at the chest, but circulates through the nerves of the nose, tongue, and glottis. It presides over speech, increases the strength of the body, improves complexion and energy, and clarifies the memory. The pervading Wind resides mainly in the heart. It distributes the vital essence by means of the circulation of the blood. In addition, it pervades the entire nervous system of the body and presides over stretching and bending the arms and legs and most of the other movements of the body such as the opening and closing of the orifices. The fire-accompanying Wind dwells mainly in the digestive tract. It circulates through the nerves of the bowels, enables the digestion of foods and beverages, separates chyle from waste, and ripens the organic components of the body. The downward-clearing Wind dwells mainly in the anal region. It circulates through the nerves of the large intestine, the sigmoid flexure, bladder, ovaries, and seminal vesicles and presides over the discharge or retention of semen, menstrual fluid, feces, and urine. See Chögyal Namkhai Norbu, *Birth, Life, and Death*.

60   Rabies for example. (ChNN)

61   These points are located four fingers, or two thumbs, below the Upper Arm Curve Points (VI.7-8).

62   Tib. *zla gzer ldang ba'i nad*. This refers to different kinds of seizures (such as epilepsy) or strokes or neurological problems and pain related to certain dates of the lunar

calendar.

63   Called Pus Points in some moxibustion manuals.

64   Corresponding to the central Posterior Lung Lobe Point (I.10).

65   The name Center of the Mirror Points (*me long dkyil gsang*) probably stems from the fact that the shoulder blade forms a nearly round shape similar to that of a Tibetan ritual mirror. (ChNN)

66   See note 53 above.

67   This type of insanity is not related to provocations, but is caused by an abnormal circulation of Wind in the body. See also Part One, note 27.

68   The symptoms of this disorder include abdominal distension, belching, sharp, sudden pain in the stomach, retching, diarrhea, and stomach rumbling.

69   See Part One, note 23.

70   The nutriment from foods does not become nutritional essence, and even if it does form, it is lost in the viscera.

71   These problems are accompanied by coughing after minor physical movements. When chronic, the symptoms of this disorder include difficult expectoration of mucus, mucus bubbling in the lungs, severe coughing at dawn and in the evening, and pain.

72   I.25, Liver Point, on the spine.

73   The symptoms of this disorder include localized pain at the lumbar region, sensation of extreme heaviness at the lumbar region, and loss of hearing.

74   I.40, Kidney Point, on the spine.

75   To find the correct spot, patients should bend their head slightly backward before measuring this point.

76   This is a severe Phlegm illness similar to the obstruction of the esophagus explained in note 10 above. (ChNN) See also note 80 below.

77   For points on the front of the body, the terms right and left refer to the patient's right and left. The sequence for treatment begins with the central point (if applicable), followed by the point on the patient's right, concluding with the point on the patient's left. See also Translator's Introduction, p. xx, and note 4 above.

78   Major and minor jugular veins (*rtse chen, rtse chung*). The minor veins at the neck are used for bloodletting in the case of viral or bacterial illnesses of the brain, lung inflammation, heart inflammation, toothache, and congestion of blood in the upper back.

79   Angina (*gag pa*), an inflammatory disease of the throat that according to Tibetan medicine also occurs in dogs and other animals and that can be contracted from animals.

80   The purpose of treating these points is to draw out a Phlegm illness that constricts the pharynx or esophagus (*bag kan mid gcus*), mentioned in relation to the Point Above the Adam's Apple, and drive it to above the tongue so as to prevent aggravation of the illness and make it curable. See also note 10 above.

81 Another point with similar benefit is the small hole between the bones. The three bones of the neck are the two parts of the collarbone and the breastbone.

82 Accompanied by difficulty in speaking.

83 See note 13 above.

84 See note 13 above.

85 The lateral points are particularly effective for these two indications.

86 Tib. *srog rlung nad*, lit. illness of the life-sustaining Wind. In this illness, the life-sustaining Wind takes a wrong course and harms the functions of the white life channel (the spinal cord). It can be caused by a diet of coarse food, strenuous activities, and other factors. This illness manifests symptoms such as agitation and restlessness, emotional instability, unhappiness and fear, confused and troubled dreams, insomnia, trembling, profuse perspiration, dizziness, yawning, difficulty with inhalation, and difficulty in swallowing food and drink. In some cases, aggravation of this illness can lead to fainting and seizures. Its symptoms are very similar to a disease known as *snying rlung* or Wind of the heart. See *gSo ba rig pa'i tshig mdzod g.yu thog dgongs rgyan*, p. 648.

87 Tib. *brang gzhun dkar nag gi mtshams* or *snying dkar nag mtshams*. Black suggests an area of thick flesh and white an area of thin flesh. The point is at the center of the imaginary line that connects the two nipples.

88 This is a symptom of a lung infection or an advanced heat disorder. It may also be associated with what in traditional Chinese medicine is referred to as true heat with false cold syndrome.

89 Tib. *lhen gsang*. These points link the esophagus and stomach. In this context *lhen* specifically refers to the mucus of the stomach that increases because of poor digestion. See *gSo ba rig pa'i tshig mdzod g.yu thog dgongs rgyan*, pp. 685-686.

90 Heartburn (*bad kan brang tsha ba*) as from gastritis.

91 Such as vomiting of blood in the case of stomach ulcers. See also note 15 above.

92 See note 15 above.

93 The Fire-Accompanying Wind Points are particularly effective for treating lack of digestive heat.

94 As in the case of women suffering from cystitis.

95 Tib. *rgyu 'or du skrangs pa*. Tibetan medicine distinguishes three types of edema: *skya rbab*, *'or*, and *dmu chu*. Early-stage edema (*sgya rbab*) shares the same primary causes with phlegm disorders in general. Its secondary condition consists in an accumulation of unassimilated nutritive essence in the liver. Failure to digest nutritive essence can be due to an incompatible diet or behavior, the consumption of foods that are difficult to digest, or stale food. In such cases, the nutritive essence accumulates, but without being assimilated cannot nourish the bodily constituents. It contributes to the production of abnormal blood and serous or lymphatic fluids that, diffused throughout the body by the Wind humor, give rise to pallor of the skin and flesh and swellings.

Symptoms include swelling of the lips, eyelids, the top of the feet, and the area of the shins; shortness of breath, palpitations, and apnea; poor digestion; pale tongue, lips, and gums; physical weakness; submerged pulse; yellowish urine; and debilitation. In the next stage (*'or*), the swelling extends to the face, chest, abdominal region, and tip of the genitals. Serous fluids are retained between the skin and flesh and the swelling in the body shifts from one side to the other, for instance when lying down. In its severe form (*dmu chu*), the serous fluids can stagnate, diffuse, exude, or erupt from degenerated tissue.

96 Tib. *long ther*. This term is variously understood by learned Tibetan doctors of the past. In his commentary to the *Four Medical Tantras* called the *Vaidurya sngon po* [Blue beryl), Desi Sangye Gyatso explains it as the *srin long* or descending part of the large intestine. See *gSo ba rig pa'i tshig mdzod g.yu thog dgongs rgyan*, p. 606.

97 This disorder presents itself through the symptom of diarrhea with bilious liquids, as in tropical diarrhea.

98 These points are considered particularly effective for treating severe edema. In this case, the term *dmu rdzing* is used rather than *dmu chu*. See also note 95 above.

99 *'Gro ba'i srog 'dzin bdud rtsi'i char rgyun* [The continuous rainfall of nectar that preserves the life of beings], by Rigdzin Changchub Dorje, Chögyal Namkhai Norbu's master. See Translator's Introduction, note 20, and Part One, p. 11 and notes 60 and 61.

100 Tib. *dmu chu*. See note 95 above.

101 See note 15 above.

102 Poisons of a cold nature (*grang dug*). In Tibetan medicine, prepared poisons are divided into poisons of a cold nature and poisons of a hot nature. Poisons prepared with minerals are of a cold nature; those whose basic ingredient is meat, resin, plants, and in particular black aconite are of a hot nature.

103 Soft bladder (*lgang snyi*) possibly refers to a distension of the bladder.

104 In some people a long crease is very evident on this part of the abdomen, hence the name of these points.

105 Tib. *mkhris pa'i nad du gyur pa*. This can be a side effect from other therapies.

106 Probably the pudendal artery.

107 This is a well-known point for increasing fertility and carrying the fetus to full term. In the context of reproductive health, moxibustion is commonly considered an effective means for turning breech babies. The relevant point, acupuncture point BL-67, is not covered in this manual. Treatment is repeated for about nine days on alternate days. See *American Journal of Chinese Medicine*, Winter, 2001, Yoichi Kanakura, et al.

108 Point III.6 (160), Central Front of the Torso.

109 Tib. *'tsho byed kyi rlung*. The term appears to be synonymous with *srog rlung*. See notes 6 and 86 above.

110 Tib. *rab rib mi gsal ba*. This is a progressive disease of the eyes that affects the liquids

of the eyes. In the first phase, the eyesight is occasionally unclear. In the second phase, looking sharply one sees objects that are near but not small, distant objects. However, one does not see clearly in the upper, lower, right, and left fields of vision (peripheral vision). When the Wind humor influences this disease, one see hairs, lights, and all forms as if they were moving. When affected by Bile, one sees flashes of light, lamps, and peacock feathers. When affected by Blood, one has a reddish vision. When affected by Phlegm, vision is obscured. In the third phase, one sees the upper but not the lower field of vision; the eyes seem veiled by a cloth. In the fourth stage, one becomes blind. See *gSo ba rig pa'i tshig mdzod g.yu thog dgongs rgyan*, pp. 419-20.

III Point III.7 (161), Central Front of the Torso.

II2 See note 13 above.

II3 Four humors (*'du ba rnam bzhi*): The three humors of Wind, Bile, and Phlegm plus Blood.

II4 The Tibetan word for collarbone (*sgrog*) means wings, as the two parts of the collarbone resemble wings.

II5 In *Cha byad dpyad*, a modern textbook of Tibetan medicine, this point is identified as *phug ron*, or Pigeon Point.

II6 Points III.9 and 10 (163 and 164), Central Front of the Torso.

II7 See note 116 above.

II8 This condition is an aggravation of the depressive syndrome. See notes 6 and 86 above.

II9 See note 53 above.

120 Points III.18 and 19 (172 and 173), Central Front of the Torso.

121 See note 99 above.

122 See Part One, note 23.

123 See note 15 above.

124 Turbid fever (*rnyog tshad*) is a disorder involving Wind, Blood, and lymph. Its primary cause is lymph. The general symptoms include a subtle and quick pulse, dark red urine, trembling heart, slight swelling of the eyelids and top of the feet, a slight cough, and pain in the upper back. It is divided into cold and hot turbid fever, each with their specific symptoms and affected areas of the body. Such a fever can lead to anemia if left untreated.

125 This point is located just below the arch of the tenth rib, where the rib curves inward. It is usually painful upon pressure.

126 See note 15 above.

127 Points III.40 and 41 (194 and 195), Central Front of the Torso.

128 Golden needle (*gser khab*): A golden needle is inserted into or positioned on the skull topped by a ball of moxa that is then lit. This form of therapy is effective for treating epilepsy and other disorders and is best used in the cold season. If performed in hot

weather, the body should be cooled an hour or so before treatment by a shower and remaining in a cool place. See Translator's Introduction, p. xviii.

129   Moxa on this point is also indicated for pain in the front or back of the head and for memory.

130   See Note 15 above.

131   As in the case of meningitis.

132   Migraine (*klad gzer*), also a name of a specific disease caused by infectious fevers that affect the brain. This disease can cause immediate death, vomiting, migraine, obfuscation of the senses, insanity, dumbness, or fainting. See *gSo ba rig pa'i tshig mdzod g.yu thog dgongs rgyan*, pp. 17-18.

133   Also indicates formation of pus in the ears.

134   See note 13 above.

135   See note 132 above.

136   See note 110 above.

137   Nest of virus and bacteria (*srin tshang*) refers to an area of the head including the temples.

138   Also sinusitis.

139   Dry irritation (*tshag skam pa*) is mainly due to Wind and Phlegm. It manifests as a dry and rough sensation in the eyes, and eyes that are particularly sensitive to cold wind.

140   Tib. *srin nad*. This problem is related to the eye's fluids. The symptoms are the formation of styes in the ocular area, itching, and an urge to rub the eyes.

141   Eye irritation (*mig tshag*) in Tibetan medicine is divided into dry irritation, humid irritation, and nagging irritation. The last can be caused by any of the four humors and has specific symptoms.

142   Tib. *rab rib kyis mig 'grib pa*. See note 110 above.

143   See note 15 above.

144   Tib. *rna ba'i 'ur zhing 'khrug pa*. The symptoms of this problem include a sensation of vacuity in the ears, severe pain in the ears, ears sensitive to cold, and pain localized in one half of the head.

145   This kind of toothache is accompanied by a lack of sensation in the gums, shooting pain in the vessels connected to the gums, and severe pain when drinking cold water or while eating cold food.

146   In this case, the person experiences severe pain when drinking hot or cold drinks or eating hot or cold food, and the toothache can vary in intensity.

147   In front of the ears where the helix joins at the temple.

148   Tib. *skya rbab*. See note 95 above.

149   Tib. *klad 'phrus rgyas pa*.

150   Tib. *gza gdon*. This is possibly the same as *gza grib*, an illness that takes its name from the beings that cause it. It is essentially a brain disorder accompanied by symptoms such as loss of speech, loss of mental functions, and fainting. See *gSo ba rig pa'i tshig mdzod g.yu*

thog dgongs rgyan, p. 536, Translator's Introduction, pp. xxii to xxiii, and note 46 above.

151 See note 47 above.

152 The point where the breath falls when the head is turned parallel to the shoulder.

153 These points are located in the indentation formed at the site of articulation when the arm is raised above the head.

154 Tib. *khrag grib*. Symptoms can include stroke, paralysis on one side, fatigue, or loss of memory and be either chronic or acute.

155 Points II.31 and II.32, or Central Shoulder Points, are referred to as Black Tip Points in Dilmar's *Me btsa'i gdams pa rgyas spros shel dkar me long* [The white crystal mirror: An extensive instruction on moxa].

156 Tib. *mig 'grib*. This can refer to external impairments such as various types of growths affecting the eyeballs or internal impairments relating to the eyeball fluid or ocular nerves as well as cataracts. Severe cases can lead to blindness.

157 Tib. *rtsa nag tu chu ser rgyug pa*. *Chuser*, translated here as lymph, is the by-product of the refinement of blood in the liver. Symptoms indicating the presence of *chuser* in the blood can include gout or skin problems such as acne or skin ulcers. See Translator's Introduction, p. xix, and Part One, note 20.

158 This point seems to correspond with TW11 on the Triple Warmer Meridian in the Chinese system.

159 Tib. *rlung 'or du skrangs pa*. See note 95 above.

160 A clarification provided by the author suggests that the pain is caused by the lymphatic disorders rather than two separate indications. Similarly, he noted a connection between gout, arthritis, and muscular cramps and spasms. See Forearm Concavity Point (VI.63-64) and note 163 below.

161 See note 160 above.

162 See Part One, note 34.

163 Tib. *chu ser phyi nang gyis sha pags gzer ba*.

164 Tib. *glo 'or*. See note 95 above.

165 Tib. *chu 'or*. See note 95 above.

166 Tib. *dbyi mig*, the articulation of the thighbone and hip bone join.

167 Horses also are subject to this problem. (ChNN)

168 Tib. *grang skran 'or du lhung ba*. See note 95 above.

169 Tib. *rne'u lhag pa'i nad*.

170 There is another point called Eye of the Crow on the torso. See III.8-10 (162-164).

171 See note 99 above.

172 Points VII.29-30 (443-444).

173 In other words, the first set of points is three thumbs below the crease at the back of the knee, the second set one thumb below that, and the third one thumb below that.

174 Tib. *chu 'or du lhung ba*. See note 95 above.

175   The tibial artery on the inside of the foot.

176   Tib. *chu ser 'or lhung*. See note 95 above.

177   Tib. *dmu chu*. See note 95 above.

178   Tib. *chu ser 'or*. See note 95 above.

179   And also without walking or straining the legs.

180   This point is also used in the case of gout and arthritis.

181   The two preceding groups of points (VII.81-82 and 83-84) are also effective for treating problems related to the eyes.

APPENDIX A

1   Most of the astrological factors referred to in this section are based on Tibetan elemental astrology (*'byung rtsis*), a complex, highly evolved system of prediction bearing few similarities to Western astrology that may well have originated in Shang Shang rather than in China as generally assumed. See Translator's Introduction, note 20. Desi Sangye Gyatso's late seventeenth-century treatise *Vaidurya dkar po*, one of the most definitive works on Tibetan elemental astrology, is available in English translation under the title *Tibetan Elemental Divination Paintings: Illuminated Manuscripts from the White Beryl* (trans. Lochen Dharmasri and Gyurme Dorje).

2   Protective energy (*bla*, pronounced la) is the base of the life force. It refers to the force of the elements in our body that protects our condition or life. This protective energy can be damaged or weakened. If this occurs, the person becomes vulnerable to negative influences and can become very weak. In this case, an ancient rite of Bön origin called recalling the protective energy (*bla 'gug*) can be performed for them. Conversely, persons with strong protective energy will be prosperous and powerful. In astrology, this is an important element along with the element of life (*srog*), body (*lus*), capacity (*dbang thang*), and fortune (*rlung rta*). Roughly speaking, life force determines the continuity, level of vital energy, and general conditions of life. Body determines health and predisposition to accidents and obstacles. Capacity determines social status and wealth, as well as the power to express and accomplish intentions. Fortune determines favorable possibilities and impediments. An individual's protective energy sustains all these factors, and especially the life force. This principle comes from the ancient Bön, where the la was conceived as a specific figure, sometimes an animal such as a dog or goat. This principle does not appear in Buddhist teachings. The place in the body where this energy resides during a particular lunar day or other period is known as the position of the protective energy (*bla gnas*).

3   In Vedic astrology, *viṣṭi*, also spelled *vishti* (Tib. *bi sthi*), is one of eleven *karaṇas*, a period of time equivalent to half a day. *Viṣṭi* is considered particularly unfavorable. See also note 27 below.

4   *Nāga Kulika* (*klu rigs ldan*): one of the eight *nāga* kings. *Nāgas* are a serpent-like class of

beings, between the animal and divine realm, that dwell in bodies of water.

5   This means that at certain times we should avoid major and risky types of external therapies such as surgical operations or moxibustion where heat is applied in direct contact with the body. For simple therapies or simple forms of moxibustion, it is not necessary to follow these precautions. However, applying the various therapies taking into consideration the position of the patient's protective energy and astrological situation could enhance the effects of the treatment.

6   The Tibetan terms for the Five Deities listed in this section are *srog lha, lus lha, dbang lha, rlung lha,* and *skyes lha,* respectively. To ascertain where an individual's Five Deities reside on the basis of his or her year of birth, one first needs to determine the elements of that individual's life force, body, capacity, fortune, and birth *mewa* (equivalent to the body *mewa*), for instance by referring to the author's book *Namkha.* The following chart, from *Tibetan Elemental Divination Paintings* (p. 63), lists correspondences between the five external elements and internal and secret locations in the body:

Phyi (External)	Nang (Internal)	gSang (Secret)
Wood	Channels	Liver
Water	Blood/Serum	Kidneys
Iron	Bones	Lungs
Earth	Flesh	Spleen
Fire	Metabolism	Heart

A simpler, albeit less specific, way to avoid the coincidence of *la* energy and the Five Deities is to refrain from treating any of the areas where *la* is transiting at a given time of the year, month, or day, as calculated by means of the charts presented in the subsequent sections of this appendix.

7   All the astrological calculations referred to in the following sections concern the aspects at the time of treatment from the perspective of the Tibetan lunar calendar. Note that the Tibetan day starts at sunrise rather than midnight. Hence, the astrological aspects relating to days of the month or days of the week should be understood as entering into effect at sunrise local time on the day in question. See Chögyal Namkhai Norbu, *Key for Consulting the Tibetan Calendar,* and the pocket calendar published each year by Shang Shung Publications.

8   A sixty-year cycle, called a *rabjung* (*rab byung*) or *metreng* (*sme phreng*), consists of five times twelve years associated with the twelve animals of the Tibetan astrological system. Each animal recurs five times linked to the five elements, wood, fire, earth, iron, and water, to make up a total of sixty years. The combination of the five elements and eight trigrams (*spar kha*) yields two sixty-year cycles or one hundred and twenty years. The system followed here starts with earth mouse and the trigram *li.* Other systems consider fire rabbit to be the starting combination for each sixty-year cycle. See note 12 below.

In the table in the original Tibetan text, the five elements (*'byung ba lnga*) are indicated by letters and the trigrams by numbers: *sha* for the wood element, *ma* for the fire element, *sa* for the earth element, *ca* for the iron element, and *cha* for the water element, 1 for *li*, 2 for *khon*, 3 for *dwa*, 4 for *khen*, 5 for *kham*, 6 for *gin*, 7 for *zin*, and 8 for *zon*.

9   Unlike the more usual classification of the elements (space, air, fire, water, and earth), in this context the element wood, having the functions of growth and movement, corresponds to the element air; the element metal or iron, having the characteristic of solidity and hardness, has the same nature as the element earth. (ChNN) See also Chögyal Namkhai Norbu, *Namkha*.

10   The 180-year cycle or *mekhor* (*sme 'khor*, lit. wheel of *mewa*) in Tibetan astrology is the cycle associated with the *sme ba* or numbers one to nine, which take three sixty-year cycles to complete.

11   Each of the three sixty-year cycles of *mewas* in a *mekhor* starts with the wood mouse in combination with a different *mewa* number (1, 4, and 7).

12   The 180-year *mekhor* cycles started in 1917 BCE with the birth of Shenrab Miwoche (*gShen rab mi bo che*) in the male wood mouse year. A more recent system considers that the sixty-year *rabjung* cycles started in the female fire rabbit year 1027 CE, when the Kalachakra Tantra was introduced to Tibet. Accordingly, the present time falls within the twenty-second *mekhor* and the seventeenth *rabjung*. See also Introduction, note 1.

13   In other words, the second time a particular animal/element combination occurs in the table of trigrams corresponds to the present seventeenth sixty-year cycle (from 1987 to 2047).

14   In our example above of the metal dragon year with the trigram *kham*, major therapies involving the genitals should have been avoided, if possible, for all patients throughout that year.

15   Zurkhar Nyamnyi Dorje (*Zur mkhar mnyam nyid rdo rje*) was a very famous doctor in twelfth-century Tibet. He was born in the earth sheep year of the seventh *rabjung* (1439/1440 CE) in a place known as Lathog Zurkhar (*Lha thog zur khar*) in eastern Dagpo (*Dwags po*).

16   Darmo (*Dar mo*), also known as Darmo Menrampa Lobsang Chödrak (*Dar mo sman rams pa blo bzang chos grags*), was the personal physician of the Fifth Dalai Lama. In charge of a traditional medical school in the Potala, he compiled various instructions on medicine in a work called *bKa' rgya ma* (*Sealed Instruction*) and many other texts, including the biographies of the younger and older Yuthog (*G.yu thog*).

17   Mipham (*Mi pham*), also known as Jamgön Ju Mipham Gyatso (*'Jam mgon 'ju mi pham rgya mtsho*, 1846-1912), was a famous Nyingma master and an expert in medicine and astrology. The Mipham system also provides correspondences for the protective energy of horses since sick horses were treated with external therapies such as bloodletting in Tibet. The position of their protective energy was taken into consideration

prior to treatment. The positions for the thirty days of the lunar month are as follows: (1) right posterior hoof sole in male horses, left posterior hoof sole in mares; (2) fatty tissue; (3) shins; (4) malleoli; (5) ankles; (6) hip sockets; (7) elbows and stifles; (8) loins; (9) soles of the front hooves; (10) soles of the front hooves; (11) fatty tissue; (12) shins of the forelegs; (13) nerves; (14) shoulders; (15) entire body; (16) neck (front and back); (17) neck (front and back); (18) along the mane; (19) nape of the neck; (20) shoulders; (21) teeth; (22) palate; (23) tongue; (24) forehead (between the eyes); (25) chest; (26) neck (front); (27) genitals; (28) testicles; (29) belly; (30) entire body.

18   *Dus 'khor bsdus rgyud* [Concise tantra of Kalachakra]. This is the extant tantra of Kalachakra. A larger one has been lost.

19   Phugpa Lhundrup Gyatso (*Phug pa lhun grub rgya mtsho*) was a celebrated scholar of astrology and author of the astronomical treatise called *Pad dkar zhal lung ma bu* [The oral instructions of Pundarika]. The Phugpa system of astronomical calculation stems from Lhundrup Gyatso and started in 1444. It is now the primary system used in preparing the Tibetan calendar.

20   *sNga 'gyur srid pa'i gter khyim* presents an interesting system of astrology of the elements found in rediscovered treasures (*gter ma*) concerning methods for overcoming various problems with mantras and rites.

21   Each solar day is assigned a number from 0 to 6. This value refers to the day of the week (Skt. *vāra*, Tib. *res gza'*) corresponding to the planet associated with that day: Saturn for Saturday, Sun for Sunday, Moon for Monday, Mars for Tuesday, Mercury for Wednesday, Jupiter for Thursday, and Venus for Friday. The Tibetan word *gza'* means planet, and the term *res gza'* literally means successive planets, indicating the cycle of planets associated with successive solar days. Saturday is indicated with 0 because in Tibet Saturday and not Sunday is considered the day of rest, a day on which it is not propitious to engage in activities such as paying wages and spending money.

22   The *sgang rtsa* is a vein used in bloodletting to treat lung fever, hoarseness, and nosebleeds. It is located four fingers below the back of the elbow.

23   The twelve periods refer to local time minus daylight saving time, if applicable.

24   The twelve periods of the day (*dus tshod bcu gnyis*) are *nam langs, nyi shar, nyi dros, nyin phyed* or *nyin gung, phyed yol, nyid myur, nyi nub, sa srod, srod 'khor, nam phyed* or *mtshan gung, gung yol*, and *tho rengs*.

25   The locations of the protective energy listed here apply only on the given day at the specified time.

26   Time of day not specified in the original Tibetan text.

27   (Tib. *mi sdug pa*). Seven are changing (Skt. *carakarana*, Tib. *'pho ba'i byed pa*): *vava* (Tib. *gdab pa*), *vālava* (Tib. *byis pa*), *kaulava* (Tib. *rigs can*), *taitila* (Tib. *til brdung*), *gara* (Tib. *khyim skyes*), *vanija* (Tib. *tshong pa*), and *viṣṭi* (Tib. *bishti*). Each of these *karanas* occupies one half

of each of the thirty lunar days in a month. Each of the fixed *karaṇas* occurs once each month around the time of the new moon. The changing *karaṇas* are spread throughout the thirty days.

28   Zodiacal astrology (*skar rtsis*) primarily refers to the astrology derived from the Kalachakra Tantra. See Translator's Introduction, note 20, and note 12 above.

29   During the periods when the *viṣṭi* and *Nāga Kulika* aspects are present and exert their negative influences, in addition to avoiding major external therapies, it is advisable not to undertake important tasks such as an inauguration.

30   This mantra is found in the discourses (sutras) of the Buddha. However, as with any mantra, to be effective the reciter must have received oral transmission from a qualified teacher. Alternatively, one can recite the following invocation, which is also from the Buddha:

> *Nyima tamche gewa yin*
> All days are virtuous,
> *Gyukar nam ni zangpo yin*
> All constellations are good.
> *Sangye nam ni nü thu che*
> The enlightened beings are powerful,
> *Drachom nam ni zagpa ze*
> All the Arhats are beyond defilements.
> *Denpai dentsig di jöpe*
> Reciting these words of truth
> *Dagchag tagtu deleg shog*
> May we always be fortunate.
> *Jaya Jaya, Sujaya*

APPENDIX B

1   Tib. *Chos rgyal nam mkha'i nor bu.*

2   At the age of two he was recognized as the reincarnation of the renowned Dzogchen master Adzom Drugpa (*A 'dzom 'brug pa*) by Palyul Karma Yangsid and Shechen Rabjam. When he was three years old, the 16th Gyalwang Karmapa recognized him as the mind incarnation of the first *dharmaraja* of Bhutan, Ngawang Namgyal.

3   Dzogchen, an abbreviation of Dzogpa Chenpo (*rDzogs pa chen po*), is a Tibetan term meaning total completion, or perfection: the original state, or condition, of every living being, whether or not they are aware of it. The knowledge of Dzogchen originated in very ancient times, but in our era it was transmitted for the first time a few centuries after Buddha Shakyamuni by Garab Dorje of Oddiyana, a region that many scholars have identified as the Swat valley in Pakistan, once a flourishing center of Buddhism. The author is one of the first Tibetan masters to have transmitted the Dzogchen

teachings in the West, first in Italy, then in numerous other countries. (See, for example, Chögyal Namkhai Norbu and Adriano Clemente, *The Supreme Source*, and Chögyal Namkhai Norbu, *Dzogchen Teachings*.)

4   Tib. *mKhyen brtse rin po che chos kyi dbang phyug* (1910-1961). The author's son, Yeshi Silvano Namkhai, was recognized as a reincarnation of Jamyang Khyentse Chökyi Wangchug and is now known as Khyentse Yeshé.

5   Tib. *rTogs ldan u rgyan bstan 'dzin* (1888-1962). See Translator's Introduction, note 19.

6   See Translator's Introduction, note 19.

7   Tib. *mKhan po mkhyen rab chos kyi 'od zer* (1889-1958).

8   Tib. *dBon stod.*

9   Khenpo Shenga (*mKhan po gzhan dga'*) was also known as Shenpen Chökyi Nangwa (*gZhan phan chos kyi snang ba*, 1871-1927).

10 Tib. *'Bo gangs dkar bshad sgrub chos kyi seng ge* (1893-1957).

11 Jamgön Kongtrul (*'Jam mgon kong strul*, 1813-1899) was a very influential and realized master, protagonist of the non-sectarian *rimé* approach in eastern Tibet.

12 *The Synthesis of the Ocean of Teachings* (*bKa' 'dus chos kyi rgya mtsho*).

13 *Il libro tibetano dei morti*, trans. by Chögyal Namkhai Norbu, p. 11.

14 See www.asia-ngo.org/en.

15 See Part One, note 3.

16 See www.shangshung.org.

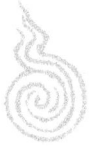

Bibliography

SOURCES IN TIBETAN

rGyud bzhi [The four medical tantras]
Full title: *bDud rtsi snying po yan lag brgyad pa gsang ba man ngag gi rgyud* [The secret oral instruction tantra on the eight limbs of the essence of nectar]

    rTsa ba'i rgyud [Root tantra]
    bShad pa'i rgyud [Explanatory tantra]
    Man ngag gi rgyud [Secret oral instruction tantra]
    Phyi ma rgyud [Last tantra]

See Part One, notes 41 and 56, for a discussion of sources of the *rGyud bzhi* and English translations published to date.

sMan dpyad zla ba'i rgyal po [The moon king]
Skt. *Somarājabhaisajyasādhanā*
Author: Uncertain. Attributed to Nāgārjuna (9th century)
Translated from the Sanskrit by Hashang Mayayana and Vairocana (other texts mention different translators)
Publisher: Mi rigs dpe skrun khang, Beijing
Date: 1985

sMan dpyad zla ba'i rgyal po [The moon king]
Version translated from the Sanskrit to Chinese and then to Tibetan (referred to here as *Somaraja*)

Pelliot tibétain 127 and *Pelliot tibétain 1044*
Two Tun-Huang manuscripts on moxibustion archived by the International Dunhuang Project, but not yet listed at http://idp.bl.uk/.

Me btsa'i gdams pa rgyas spros shel dkar me long [The white crystal mirror: An extensive instruction on moxa]
Author: Dilmar Geshe Tenzin Phuntshog (*Dil dmar dge bshes bstan 'dzin phun tshogs*; 1672-?)

'Gro ba'i srog 'dzin bdud rtsi'i char rgyun [The continuous rainfall of nectar that preserves the life of beings]
Author: Rigdzin Changchub Dorje (*Rig 'dzin byang chub rdo rje*, 1826-1961)

Tshe rig rgyud 'bum bye ba'i yang bcud zur rgyan nyer mkho dpag bsam ljon shing bzang po [The excellent wish-fulfilling tree: An indispensable ornament of the quintessence of myriad treatises on the art of healing]
Author: Khyungchen Pungri Khyungtrul Jigme Namkhai Dorje Yungdrung Gyaltsan (*Khyung sprul 'jigs med nam mkha'i rdo rje gyung drung rgyal mtshan*, 1897-1955)

Vaidurya sngon po [Blue beryl]
Author: Desi Sangye Gyatso (*sDe srid sangs rgyas rgya mtsho*; 1653-1705)

Vaidurya dkar po [White beryl]
Author: Desi Sangye Gyatso
(See below for English edition)

gSo ba rig pa'i tshig mdzod g.yu thog dgongs rgyan [Ornament of Yutog's mind: A dictionary of healing arts]
Author: Wangdu (*dBang 'dus*)
Publisher: Mi rigs dpe skrun khang, Beijing
Date: 1982

bKa' phreng mun sel sgron me [Garland of teachings: Lamp that dispels the darkness]
Author: Darmo Menrampa (*Dar mo sman rams pa blo bzang chos grags*; 1638-1710)

bLa gnas brtsi ba'i zin bris gsal ba'i me long [The clear mirror: Notes on calculating the location of protective energy]
Author: Nyamnid Dorje (*mNyam nyid rdo rje*; 1439-1475)

rTsis skor nor bu'i phreng ba [Jewel garland of astrology]
Author: Jamgön Ju Mipham Gyatso (*'Jam mgon 'ju mi pham rgya mtsho*; 1846-1912)

Cha byad dpyad [Medical instruments]
Editor: Lobzang Damchö (*Blo bzang dam chos*)
Publisher: Mi rigs dpe skrun khang, Beijing
Date: 2004

SOURCES IN ENGLISH

Chögyal Namkhai Norbu. *The Necklace of Gzi: A Cultural History of Tibet*. Dharamsala: Information Office of HH the Dalai Lama, 1980.

————. *The Necklace of Gzi: On the History and Culture of Tibet*, Arcidosso: Shang Shung Publications, 2004.

————, trans. *Il libro tibetano dei morti*. Rome: Newton Compton, 1983.

Chögyal Namkhai Norbu and Adriano Clemente. *The Supreme Source*. Ithaca: Snow Lion Publications, 1999.

Chögyal Namkhai Norbu. *Namkha*. Arcidosso: Shang Shung Publications, 1999.

————. *The Practice of Tibetan Kunye Massage*. Arcidosso: Shang Shung Publications, 2003.

————. *Key for Consulting the Tibetan Calendar*. Arcidosso: Shang Shung Publications, 2003.

————. *Dzogchen Teachings*. Ithaca: Snow Lion Publications, 2006.

————. *Yantra Yoga: The Tibetan Yoga of Movement*. Ithaca: Snow Lion Publications, 2008.

————. *Birth, Life, and Death*. Arcidosso: Shang Shung Publications, 2008.

————. *The Light of Kailash: A History of Zhang Zhung and Tibet*, vol. I: *The Early Period*. Trans. Donatella Rossi. Arcidosso: Shang Shung Publications, 2009.

————. *Zhang Zhung: Images from a Lost Kingdom*. Arcidosso: Shang Shung Publications, 2010.

————. *Rainbow Body: The Life and Liberation of Togden Ugyen Tendzin*. Arcidosso: Shang Shung Publications, 2010.

Desi Sangye Gyatso. *Tibetan Elemental Divination Paintings: Illuminated Manuscripts from the White Beryl*. Original title: *Vaidurya dkar po*. Trans. Lochen Dharmasri and Gyurme Dorje. London: Sam Fogg Ltd and John Eskenazi Ltd, 2001.

————. *A Mirror of Beryl: A Historical Introduction to Tibetan Medicine*. Original title: *Vaidurya sngon po*. Trans. Gavin Kilty. Library of Tibetan Classics. Somerville: Wisdom Publications, 2010.

Minyag Gonpo. *The Incarnation from White Glacier Mountain: The Biography of Gangkar Rinpoche*. Trans. S. Brinson Aldridge. West Conshohocken: Infinity Publishing, 2008.

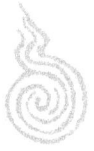

Indications Index

This index lists illnesses that can be treated with moxibustion along with the respective points suitable for treatment. The points are identified with the Roman/Arabic numeral code used in Part Two. The Roman numerals represent the seven areas of the body and the Arabic numerals designate consecutive sequences within each of the seven areas of the body. Refer to the General Index for conditions mentioned outside of the Compendium of Points and Indications.

I: Points Along the Spine
II: Points on the Lateral Back
III: Points on the Central Front of the Torso
IV: Points on the Lateral Front of the Torso
V: Points on the Head
VI: Points on the Arms
VII: Points on the Legs

Abdomen
- and liver, swelling of VII.31-32
- cold sensation in, accompanied by poor digestion I.16-18

Abdominal distension III.26-28, III.32-34, III.39
- and empty rumblings when exposed to cold I.47-49
- and pain I.25-27
- and pain caused by spleen disorders III.29-31
- and rumbling IV.29-30
- and rumbling, frequent III.40-41
- and rumbling in the small and large intestines I.44-46
- beginning in the afternoon III.29-31
- frequent, and sensation of fullness I.31-33

Abdominal noises (see also Abdominal distension)
- and rumbling I.31-33, III.42-44

caused by pulmonary diseases
I.10-12

Ureteral trauma II.71-72

Urethra
* burning sensation at the tip of
I.40-42, I.44-46, I.56-58
* pain at the tip of III.48-50

Urinary bladder
* tumors and other illnesses of I.44-
46

Urination
* frequent I.40-42, I.56-58, I.62-64,
III.48-50

Urine, blood or pus in (see Kidney
disorders)

Urine retention I.40-42, I.47-49,
III.42-44, III.58-60, VII.65-66,
VII.69-70
* and constipation I.50-52
* and frequent urination III.64-65
* and internal swellings, after
childbirth (Wind-related) III.38
* and loss of nutritional essence in
women III.35-37
* and related pain and discomfort
III.45-47
* or frequent urination when exposed
to cold I.50-52, I.53-55, III.51-53

Uterine illnesses III.54, III.48-50

Uterine pain III.48-50

Uterus
* tumors of I.37-39

Vagina
* aching or swelling at the opening
of I.56-58

Vaginal discharge III.58-60

Vaginal fluids
* accumulation or discharge of
I.50-52

Vaginal labia
* swelling of III.63

Vascular conditions VII.41-46
* and neurological conditions, caused
by contamination II.31-40
* Wind-related I.69-71, VII.41-46

Vascular system
* abnormal presence of lymph in
VI.17-22
* Bile flowing into I.4-6
* Bile spreading or diffusing into I.4-6

Vertigo (see also Dizziness)
* and sensation as if the body were
sinking VII.61-62
* and sensation of falling over when
leaning V.76
* and sensation that the head is
spinning during movement V.76

Viral or bacterial illnesses I.37-39,
II.63-64, III.55-57
* aggravation of II.65-66
* of the blood I.78-80
* of the brain V.1
* of the head I.66-68

Viral or bacterial infections III.48-50

Viral or bacterial kidney disorders
II.71-72, II.73-74

Viruses or bacteria
* associated with Wind disorders,
nasal congestion caused by I.66-68
* in the blood, concentration or
dispersion of V.2-3
* white and black, illnesses caused by

Vision (see also Eyesight)
* impaired IV.1-2, V.6-7, V.12,
V.19-20, V.24, V.76, VII.23-24
* severely impaired V.21-22
* unclear I.28-30, V.76

Vital essence

preservation of I.37-39

Voice (see also Speech)
- loss of V.4-5
- quavering III.6

Vomit (see also Retching)
- inability to III.6

Vomiting I.13-15, I.34-36, II.61-62, III.4-5, III.26-28, III.29-31, IV.3-4, IV.15-16, VI.37-38
- Phlegm-related IV.23-28
- bile I.28-30
- of blood, caused by liver illness I.22-24, I.25-27, III.32-34

Waist (see also Lumbar region)
- pain in, when bending forward or backward IV.19-20

Warts
- and other skin problems VI.49-50

Waterborne illnesses (see Pain or malaise from drinking certain types of water)

Weakness and pain
- caused by cold illnesses III.38

Weight loss and physical lightness
- promotion of I.37-39

Wind and Bile disorders
- combined I.78-80

Wind and Blood disorders (see also Dazed feeling, Eyes, Heart, Upper back)
- combined I.72-74, V.24
- combined, caused by the five types of Wind II.41-48

Wind and Phlegm disorders (see also Eyeballs)
- combined, head problems caused by I.13-15
- combined, or an abnormal blood condition, illnesses related to V.76

Wind disorders I.4-6, I.7-9 (see also Downward-clearing Wind, Life-sustaining Wind, and individual indications)
- affecting the joints VII.3-4, VII.15-18, VII.59-60
- affecting the coronaries, insanity caused by I.1-3
- arising after a fever II.63-64
- after childbirth I.50-52, III.39, III.51-53
- caused by contamination V.79, VI.35-36, VI.39-48, VI.63-64
- in general; problems in the inner and outer parts of the body caused by minor Wind disorders or scattered Wind II.41-48
- minor, or scattered Wind, intercostal pain resulting from III.25
- minor, or scattered Wind, problems in the inner and outer parts of the body caused by II.41-48
- pain caused by I.25-27
- severe illnesses related to I.62-64

Wind humor
- affecting the upper body III.11-13, III.14-16
- of a cold nature I.47-49, I.62-64, III.40-41, IV.19-20
- of a cold nature, affecting the lower body III.48-50
- of a cold nature, illnesses related to I.7-9
- of a cold nature, increase of I.37-39, III.32-34
- of a cold nature, increase of, in the womb I.43

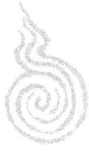

General Index

The General Index predominantly contains references to sections of the manual outside of the Compendium of Points. The majority of specific indications are listed in the Indications Index, which is a comprehensive listing of all indications included in the Compendium of Points. Indications not referred to directly in the Compendium of Points are included in the General Index. Tibetan terms given in Wylie transliteration are alphabetized by first letter, even if it is not the root letter.

www.ingramcontent.com/pod-product-compliance
Lightning Source LLC
Chambersburg PA
CBHW080931240326

41458CB00141B/3085